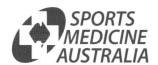

Sports Medicine Australia (SMA) was founded in 1963 and is a national multidisciplinary organisation of professionals committed to working together to enhance the health of all Australians through safe participation in sport, recreation and physical activity. SMA is Australia's peak advisory body on all medical and health issues for active people – from weekend enthusiasts of all ages through to elite level competition.

SMA has a broad membership of sports medicine and health professionals, researchers and academics, sports trainers, sporting clubs and community members, all of whom share an interest in safe sport and physical activity. SMA's multidisciplinary approach to sports medicine and science has played an important part in the success of Australia's athletes and sporting teams, and SMA members' shared knowledge and skills play an important part in keeping all Australians active and healthy. SMA members can be found at every level of physical activity and sport from elite competition to grass-roots participation.

SMA provides expert information, advice and commentary on issues such as government policy and funding for sports medicine and community activity through to sports health, gender equity, participation of the aged in sport, safe sport for children and drugs in sport problems. SMA also plays an active role in educating professionals and sports-minded community members and in assisting all active people to achieve optimal benefits from their exercise, activity and competition.

http://sma.org.au

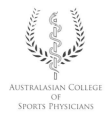

AUSTRALASIAN COLLEGE
OF
SPORTS PHYSICIANS

The Australasian College of Sports Physicians (ACSP) is the professional body representing sports physicians in both Australia and New Zealand. Sports physicians are committed to excellence in the practice of medicine as it applies to all aspects of physical activity. Safe and effective sporting performance at all levels is a major focus. Alongside this is the increasing recognition of the importance of exercise in the prevention and treatment of common and often serious medical conditions, such as arthritis, heart disease, diabetes and many cancers. The ACSP was founded by a dedicated group of like-minded practitioners in 1985.

http://www.acsp.org.au

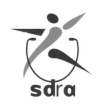

sdra

Sports Doctors Australia (SDrA) is a professional society of medical practitioners dedicated to promoting and communicating the highest levels of knowledge, research and education in sports medicine. It consists of doctors from a wide area of specialties including general practice, emergency medicine, rehabilitation medicine and orthopaedics. Many have postgraduate degrees in sports medicine and have vast experience as team doctors.

http://www.sportsdoctors.com.au/

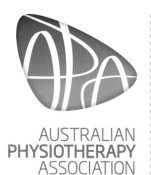

AUSTRALIAN
PHYSIOTHERAPY
ASSOCIATION

Australian Physiotherapy Association (APA)—Sport Physiotherapy Group
The Australian Physiotherapy Association (APA) is the peak body representing the interests of Australian physiotherapists and their patients. The APA is a national organisation with specialty subgroups including Sports Physiotherapy Australia (SPA). Members of SPA have experience and knowledge of the latest evidence-based practice, skilled assessment and diagnosis of sports injuries, and use effective 'hands-on' management techniques to assist recovery and prevent injury.

http://www.physiotherapy.asn.au

Sports Dietitians Australia (SDA) is a national organisation of qualified sports dietitians. SDA is leading the promotion of healthy eating to enhance the performance of all Australians whatever their level of physical activity. Sports dietitians assist Australians to make healthier food choices by providing accurate nutrition information based on scientific principles. Sports dietitians work with elite and recreational athletes, sporting clubs, active children and anyone whose nutrition needs play an important part in achieving their health and activity goals.

http://www.sportsdietitians.com.au

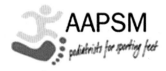

The Australasian Academy of Podiatric Sports Medicine (AAPSM) encourages research in the areas of musculoskeletal pathomechanics, biomechanical analysis and orthotic control as applied to the athletic community.

The AAPSM also encourages accumulation of statistics in the area of sports medicine in order to develop sound methods of prevention and treatment of sports injuries. The AAPSM participates in the annual Conference of Science and Medicine in Sport to disseminate current knowledge to the profession, allied professions and those engaged in the treatment of amateur, professional or individual athletics.

http://www.aapsm.org.au

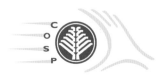

College of Sport and Exercise Psychologists

The APS College of Sport and Exercise Psychologists is a professional association of psychologists who are interested in how participation in sport, exercise and physical activity may enhance personal development and wellbeing throughout the life span.

The College of Sport and Exercise Psychologists develops and safeguards the standards of practice and supervised experience. It sets the quality of service in sport and exercise psychology and advises and makes recommendations regarding the education and training of sport and exercise psychologists.

http://www.groups.psychology.org.au/csep/

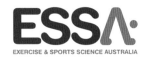

Exercise Sports Science Australia

Founded in 1991, Exercise & Sports Science Australia (ESSA), formerly known as the Australian Association for Exercise and Sports Science (AAESS), is a professional organisation that is committed to establishing, promoting and defending the career paths of tertiary-trained exercise and sports science practitioners. ESSA's vision is to enhance the health and performance of all Australians through the support of exercise and sports science professionals.

http://www.essa.org.au

SPORTS MEDICINE
For Sports Trainers

TENTH EDITION

Sports Medicine Australia

SPORTS MEDICINE
For Sports Trainers

TENTH EDITION

Sports Medicine Australia

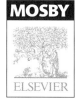
MOSBY
ELSEVIER

Sydney   Edinburgh   London   New York   Philadelphia   St Louis   Toronto

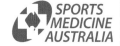
SPORTS MEDICINE AUSTRALIA

Mosby

is an imprint of Elsevier

Elsevier Australia. ACN 001 002 357
(a division of Reed International Books Australia Pty Ltd)
Tower 1, 475 Victoria Avenue, Chatswood, NSW 2067

National Library of Australia Cataloguing-in-Publication Data

---

Sports medicine for sports trainers / Sports Medicine Australia.

10th ed.
9780729541541 (pbk.)
Includes index.

Sports medicine–Handbooks, manuals, etc.
Athletic trainers–Training of–Australia.
Sports injuries–Handbooks, manuals, etc.
Sports–Safety measures–Handbooks, manuals, etc.

Sports Medicine Australia.

617.1027

Publisher: Melinda McEvoy
Developmental Editor: Amanda Simons
Project Coordinators: Natalie Hamad and Nayagi Athmanathan
Edited by Linda Littlemore
Proofread by Tim Learner
Indexed by Robert Swanson
Illustrations by Michael Towey
Photography by Chris Canham Photography
Cover and internal design by George Creative
Typeset by Toppan Best-set Premedia Limited
Printed in China by 1010 Printing Int'l Ltd.

FOREWORD

Sports Medicine Australia is a national multidisciplinary organisation of professionals committed to enhancing the health of all Australians through safe participation in sport, recreation and physical activity.

One of the key reasons for the formation of Sports Medicine Australia was to ensure athletes are able to access the best available sports medicine care. Over many years sports trainers, along with many other sports medicine professionals, have continued to play a major role in athlete care at all levels of sport. This is particularly so in community sporting settings where the sports trainer is often the first respondent to an athlete injury and a key part of the sports medicine referral network.

Athlete care, including preparation for competition, injury treatment and injury management, is as important today as it has ever been and sports trainers continue to be an integral part of the sports medicine team at all levels of sport.

Sports Medicine Australia, through the Safer Sport Program, has for many years been the primary training body for sports trainers in Australia. *Sports Medicine for Sports Trainers* has long been the leading reference text in the education of sports trainers in Australia. It has been specifically developed to incorporate the fundamental skills and knowledge required in the role of a sports trainer based on the latest sports medicine research and contemporary best practice. This 10th edition of *Sports Medicine for Sports Trainers* continues this tradition.

Thank you for participating in this important training program.

Dr Rob Reid
Safer Sport Delegate
Sports Medicine Australia National Board

EDITOR'S NOTE AND ACKNOWLEDGEMENTS

The Tenth Edition of *Sports Medicine for Sports Trainers* builds on the previous editions by once again compiling evidence-based information sourced from the latest available scientific information and peer-reviewed guidelines. One of the key changes is that the Tenth Edition now also incorporates the Sports Medicine Australia (SMA) Level 1 and Level 2 Sports Trainer curriculums. This has resulted in several new sections, including an introduction to basic sports massage, and more comprehensive coverage of topics such as sports taping to reflect the curriculum requirements for SMA Level 2 Sports Trainer accreditation. Another change is that the chapter on sports injury prevention has been substantially modified to reflect a focus on the concept of sports injury prevention being a system comprised of a collection of inter-related processes that includes, but is not limited to, warm-up programs and protective equipment alone.

A hierarchy of evidence was used in determining what should be included in the content of the Tenth Edition. Whenever possible, information was based on peak or expert advisory body guidelines, such as the Australian Resuscitation Council crisis management guidelines, or on expert consensus group guidelines, such as in the revised section on the management of concussion in sport. For topics where such clear guidelines do not exist the text was updated based on expert input from a range of sports medicine health professionals and other industry experts who provided information on the latest best practice approaches used in the field of sports medicine, and further drawing when possible on the most recent peer-reviewed scientific publications.

Given the broad range of topics covered in this book, input was required from a diverse range of individuals and organisations with expertise in the areas covered. This being the case and also taking into consideration that the Tenth Edition does represent an ongoing evolution since the introduction many years ago of the SMA Safer Sport Program and the resultant First Edition, it is impossible to list all who have contributed to this latest edition.However, SMA would like to especially acknowledge:

The editors, authors and contributors to all previous editions and other publications utilised in the SMA Safer Sport Program and, in particular, Dean Dudley who edited the Ninth Edition

The Sports Medicine Australia Board of Directors, State Branches, Discipline Groups, Executive Management Group and Education Managers Group for providing direction, suggestions, corrections, and additions to the text

Dr Rob Reid, who provided substantial technical direction, content and editorial assistance

The SMA ACT Branch for assistance in organising the main photo shoot, and also to Daramalan College Canberra for hosting this.

Asics Australia

Beiersdorf Australia Ltd

Mark Brown, Editor

PICTURE CREDITS

CONTENTS

Contents

INTRODUCTION

About this book

This book has been developed primarily as a reference text for the Sports Medicine Australia Safer Sport Program Sports Trainer courses and provides introductory information related to the range of competencies required of people operating as sports trainers. However, it can also be used in conjunction with other secondary, tertiary and vocational health-related courses including units of competency from the Australian SIS 10 Sport, Fitness and Recreation Training Package. Additionally, it will also be of interest and use as a reference for all people interested in safe sport and physical activity.

Consistent with the breadth of the role of the sports trainer, the book covers several areas and draws upon expertise and research provided by a wide range of health professionals, scientists and other practitioners in the areas of sports medicine and sports science.

Sports Medicine Australia Safer Sport Program

The SMA Safer Sport Program was developed by SMA with the philosophy of providing a safe environment for all Australians who engage in sport and to maximise participation in physical activity. The Safer Sport Program aims to achieve this by providing courses for all people involved or interested in sport or physical activity with a distinct emphasis on gaining practical skills, such as sports injury prevention, immediate injury management and crisis management techniques, that can be used in a sporting environment.

The training material in the Safer Sport Program courses has been developed by SMA's professional members from the most recent available evidence and research in sports medicine and sports science. The Safer Sport Program courses include Sports Medicine Awareness, Sports First Aid, Level 1 Sports Trainer, Level 2 Sports Trainer and other courses developed to improve prevention and management of injuries and medical conditions potentially associated with participation in sport and physical activity.

Successful completion of the SMA Safer Sport Program Level 1 and Level 2 Sports Trainer courses entitles the participant to accreditation as an SMA Sports Trainer. SMA Sports Trainer accreditation is recognised by most Australian sporting organisations for the provision of first contact sports medicine services.

The SMA Safer Sport Program and the Australian Qualifications Framework

The Australian Qualifications Framework (AQF) is the national policy for regulated qualifications in Australian education and training. It incorporates the qualifications from each education and training sector into a single comprehensive national qualifications framework.

AQF qualifications certify the knowledge and skills that a person has achieved through study, training, work and life experience. An AQF qualification is the result of an accredited complete program of learning that leads to formal certification that a graduate has achieved learning outcomes as described in the AQF. An AQF qualification is recognised throughout Australia and also by some other countries. For more information about the AQF visit the website (www.aqf.edu.au).

AQF qualifications are classified according to a system of 10 levels ranging from Certificate I (Level 1) to a Doctoral Degree (Level 10). An SMA Sports Trainer accreditation represents training and competencies of a Certificate III standard under the AQF. Sports Medicine Australia and many SMA training partners award Statements of Attainment and provide recognition of prior learning (RPL) for certain SMA Safer Sport Program qualifications.

AQF qualifications are grouped by industry sectors into several different training packages. Each qualification in the training packages includes a prescribed number and types of units of competency to achieve the award of that particular qualification. The SMA Sports Trainer accreditation is aligned with units of competency from the SIS 10 Sport, Fitness and Recreation Training Package, in particular units from the SIS30810 Certificate III Sports Trainer qualification.

Recognition of prior learning (RPL)

The SMA recognition of prior learning (RPL) process recognises the competencies that may already have been achieved either through other courses or training you have participated in or from work or life experience. If what you have learned at work or elsewhere is relevant to the course or prerequisites for a course, you may not have to do those parts of the course again.

Applying for recognition of prior learning

There is a specific process to determine whether you can be granted exemption from units of competency or from prerequisites for enrolling in a course. If you apply for recognition of prior learning or current competency, you will be given the course 'learning outcomes' and 'performance criteria' of the unit(s) of competency and asked to document details of your experience to allow comparison of your knowledge and skills against the course competencies. In most cases, you will then be asked to attend an interview with course and RPL experts. Before the interview you will be provided with information on what kinds of information or any other help you may need at the interview as well as details on how you might be assessed. You may have a friend, relative or expert join you at the interview. At the interview, the interviewers may help you complete your application form if necessary.

If your application is successful, you will not be required to do certain parts of your course or will be granted prerequisites. In some cases, before a decision is made on your application you may be asked to provide extra information or you may ask to provide additional information to assist in the assessment of your application.

If you are interested in more information regarding this process, contact your local SMA state/territory branch.

Career prospects

Sports trainers can seek employment on either a voluntary or paid basis and work at all levels of sport in Australia from amateur to professional sport. Especially at the community level, sports trainers are an integral part of sport in Australia and have a vital role in ensuring that sport and physical activity are safer and more enjoyable for all who are involved.

There is an increasing number of paid and career sports trainers who receive remuneration for their time working with athletes and assisting with the provision of sports medicine coverage services, both directly for sporting clubs and at sporting events. For more information about becoming involved in this type of work, contact your local SMA branch.

Chapter One

THE SPORTS TRAINER IN ACTION

LEARNING OUTCOMES

1 Explain the operations expected of a sports trainer and the contexts in which they should be applied
2 Describe the accepted roles and responsibilities of a sports trainer
3 Demonstrate accepted safety and privacy practices
4 Detail ways of developing positive relationships with health care professionals
5 Demonstrate effective communication with athletes, coaches, parents and health care professionals
6 Detail professional development programs and options
7 Describe the components and processes necessary to establish a fair and equitable sporting environment
8 Demonstrate a range of emergency hand signals
9 Describe ethical and legal issues related to the activities of a sports trainer
10 Demonstrate effective communication skills between injured athletes and support staff
11 Demonstrate safe handling, maintenance and storage protocols of sports medicine equipment
12 Describe methods of accurately recording the details of an injured athlete

ASSESSMENT OF OUTCOMES

Underpinning knowledge

Oral or written questions may be asked relating to the conduct and behaviour of sports trainers with respect to their accepted roles and responsibilities. You may also be asked to complete an online learning task related to equality in sport and submit copies of completed online tasks.

Practical demonstration

You may be asked to show how you would document the treatment of your athletes or manage their personal medical information. You may also be required to identify specific items of sports medicine equipment and describe their purpose.

Scenario

You may be asked to locate sports medicine equipment and use it in simulated emergency situations. You may also be asked to document and record athlete assessments and treatments.

Introduction

This chapter describes the role of the sports trainer as well as the relationships between the sports trainer and sporting organisations and Sports Medicine Australia (SMA). It is essential that all candidates have a clear understanding of the role, relationships and responsibilities of a sports trainer. The sports trainer must be able to:

- understand and operate within their scope of practice
- adhere to accepted safety and privacy practices
- contribute to a safe, fair and equitable sporting environment
- communicate effectively with athletes, coaches, parents and health care professionals
- work collaboratively with, and refer appropriately to, health care professionals
- appreciate ethical issues surrounding first aid and sports medicine
- handle, maintain and store sports medicine equipment
- identify continuing education and development options.

What is a sports trainer?

Sports trainers are members of the sports medicine team who are able to provide basic injury prevention and management techniques as well as assist in improving athletic performance. Sports trainers provide a crucial link between the athlete, coach and sports medicine health professionals. They are often the first to respond when an athlete requires assistance with an injury or medical condition; however, their role is more comprehensive than simply providing first aid only. The sports trainer's role includes:

- implementing appropriate injury prevention protocols
- preparing players for competition
- providing the appropriate immediate management of injuries
- providing immediate crisis management of severe injuries
- informed referral of injuries to a more qualified health professional for further advice and management
- working in conjunction with health professionals, such as physiotherapists or doctors, to ensure a safe return to play for injured players
- educating players and coaching staff in relation to return to play principles.

Applying these skills improves the likelihood of a good outcome for anyone who has a sports-related injury or illness.

The role of the sports trainer varies depending on the type and level of the team. With high level sports teams, sports trainers usually work in conjunction with health professionals, such as doctors and physiotherapists. However, in community level sport,

the sports trainer is likely to be the only person present with any medical training.

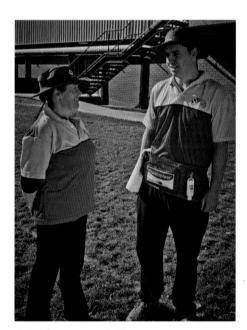

Figure 1.1 The sports trainer

Under the Sports Medicine Australia Safer Sport Program, sports trainers can be accredited as either a Level 1 or Level 2 Sports Trainer.

The requirements to achieve accreditation as an SMA Level 1 Sports Trainer include:

- having a current Apply First Aid Certificate, or equivalent
- having a current Cardiopulmonary Resuscitation (CPR) Certificate
- completion of the SMA Safer Sport Program Level 1 Sports Trainer course, or equivalent.

Accredited Level 2 Sports Trainers are expected to be able to provide appropriate care of athletes to a more advanced standard than Level 1 Sports Trainers. The requirements for SMA Level 2 accreditation include:

- fulfilment of the accreditation criteria for a Level 1 Sports Trainer
- completion of the SMA Safer Sport Program Level 2 Sports Trainer course, or equivalent.

Sports trainers can operate as volunteers or they may work for remuneration in return for their time and expertise. In either case, sports trainers should be aware of, and always operate in accordance with, the Sports Trainer Code of Ethics, which is discussed later in this chapter.

The sports trainer will be expected to provide support and advice to a range of people involved in sport, including amateur and professional athletes, their coaches, managers and other sports administrators. The sports trainer's role may therefore include tasks related to:

- athlete health and wellbeing
- athlete performance
- athlete education and development
- legal documentation and responsibility
- budgeting and acquisition of medical equipment and consumables
- liaison with sporting officials and administration decision makers
- first aid and emergency care of athletes.

Sports trainers and the law

Although sports trainers are not registered or regulated health practitioners under Australian law, the role of the sports trainer is still subject to some legal restrictions. Therefore, sports trainers need to be familiar with their legal obligations.

There are some legal principles that all sports trainers should understand and be careful to comply with, including:

1 consent
   a informed consent
   b implied consent
2 duty of care
3 negligence
4 scope of practice
5 restricted practices.

Consent

The principle of consent recognises that all athletes have the right to accept or refuse treatment or assistance. There are two main types of consent sports trainers need to be aware of:

1 Informed consent – sometimes also known as actual consent or express consent. For informed consent, the athlete or the parent/

guardian specifically gives the sports trainer permission to help or render assistance. To gain a proper informed consent, it is necessary to explain to the athlete the likely benefits of the suggested treatment or intervention, as well as the possible risks and the alternative options available to them.

2 Implied consent – consent not actually granted by the person but implied from their actions or silence. It is based on what a reasonable person would usually expect to be done in the circumstances. For example, in an emergency situation, an unconscious athlete's consent to assistance is implied.

Duty of care

Duty of care describes the duty of all people to take reasonable care to act in a way that will not cause harm to a person under their care. It also includes the obligation to provide assistance, if possible, but does not oblige a person to provide assistance if doing so would at the same time put them at risk.

As part of their role to provide assistance and emergency care to athletes, a sports trainer usually has an implied duty of care to provide assistance as effectively as they can within the limitations of their scope of practice and without putting themselves at risk. As part of the their duty of care, once they have started to provide assistance the sports trainer should stay with the person requiring assistance until more qualified health care professionals arrive.

Negligence

Negligence as a legal concept usually refers to harm caused by carelessness or lack of skill rather than intentional harm. To establish whether an act was negligent, a court must first be satisfied that the defendant owed a duty of care to the complainant. If a duty of care was owed, then the court must decide:

- was harm foreseeable?
- what is the usual practice or standard of care?
- was it likely that harm would occur as a result of the action actually undertaken?

Scope of practice

Scope of practice refers to the role, responsibilities and range of tasks that are both legally and ethically appropriate for a sports trainer to undertake. The sports trainer's scope of practice is determined by what they are legally allowed to do, their level of training and their ethical and contractual obligations. In other words, their scope of practice may vary according to the role they have been employed or contracted to undertake, but can never exceed those restricted under law. In addition, a sports trainer's scope of practice is restricted to encompass only skills they have acquired as a result of their training, and is further restricted to only those activities allowable under both the Sports Trainer Code of Ethics and their contract of service.

Restricted practices

Restricted practices are medical procedures or techniques that are specifically restricted by law. These techniques can only be used by registered health professionals who have authority under the law to do so, such as doctors, physiotherapists, podiatrists and the other health professions registered by the Australian Health Practitioner Regulation Agency. Examples of restricted practices that are illegal for sports trainers to undertake include surgical and dental procedures, prescription and supply of scheduled medications and spinal manipulation or adjustments.

If sports trainers perform, or attempt to perform, any restricted practices limited to registered health professionals, they may have legal action taken against them, including prosecution. Their sports trainer accreditation with SMA may also be cancelled.

Insurance

Sports trainers should ensure that they have appropriate professional indemnity insurance coverage. Sometimes, they may be covered by insurance held by the sports club or organisation they are working for, especially if they are working as volunteers. Some sports insurance policies specifically do not cover medical procedures and, accordingly, will not include work done by sports trainers; others do not cover people working for remuneration.

Therefore, it is recommended that sports trainers consider obtaining appropriate personal professional indemnity insurance, especially if they are working for more than one club or sporting organisation.

Safety, health and wellbeing

Sporting environments can potentially include hazards and conditions that, although unusual and unlikely, can lead to personal injury, illness or even death. These hazards can pose a significant risk to the safety, health and wellbeing of athletes, officials, supporters and sports trainers.

The following sections examine some areas in which sports trainers can identify and minimise the risk of an accident or prevent an incident from occurring that may harm the sports trainer, the athletes, the spectators or others at sporting venues and events.

Physical health and fitness

It is essential that sports trainers maintain a reasonable level of physical fitness as the work that

many of them undertake can be physically demanding, especially in an emergency. Regular physical exercise and an appropriate diet help sports trainers to not only avoid injury and illness but may also improve their ability to provide assistance to others. Sports trainers should consider consulting an appropriate health professional, such as an exercise physiologist, physiotherapist, certified fitness instructor or personal trainer, for advice on a suitable exercise program for their personal circumstances to maximise their personal fitness.

Sports trainers should also be role models for positive physical health and fitness. Sports trainers are in a position to positively model appropriate behaviour with regard to exercise and diet, as well as drug, alcohol and tobacco use, to the athletes under their care.

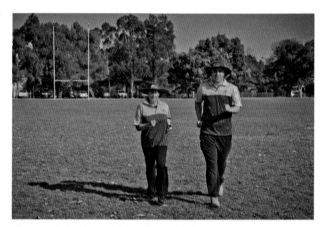

Figure 1.2 Physical health and fitness is important for sports trainers

Sun protection

Working outdoors for an extended time often exposes sports trainers to long periods of ultraviolet (UV) radiation. Exposure to UV radiation is a major cause of sunburn, premature skin ageing, cataracts and several forms of skin cancer.

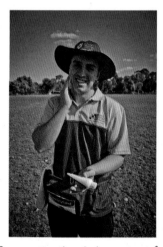

Figure 1.3 Sun protection is important for sports trainers and athletes

Sports trainers can prevent damage to themselves and their athletes by adhering to the following guidelines:

- Limit exposure to the sun, especially during the hottest parts of the day, or when the sun is at its highest, which is usually between 10 a.m. and 3 p.m.
- Wear sun protective clothing, such as collared long-sleeve shirts, hats or sun visors and eye protection.
- Wear high sun protection factor (SPF) sunscreens (SPF 30+ or higher). Ensure that sunscreen is applied to all sun-exposed skin.
- Provide shelter or shade for break periods in play and provide constant shade for officials, coaches and non-active athletes where possible.

Obstructed, slippery or untidy working areas

The working area or medical room and areas set aside for athletes should be kept clean and free of clutter. Obstructions, tripping hazards and slippery surfaces can create injury hazards to all present.

Untidy working areas may also make it harder to locate important equipment promptly and prevent a quick and appropriate response to an emergency.

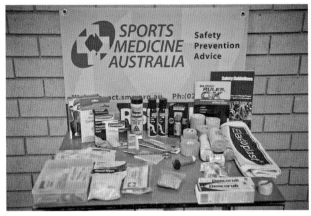

Figure 1.4 A tidy work area improves efficiency and safety

Serviceability of and faulty sports medicine equipment and incorrect storage

Missing, damaged or faulty sports medicine equipment can potentially put an athlete's life in danger. Regular stocktakes and inspection of equipment prior to providing sports training services is an important part of the sports trainers' role.

The sports trainer should ensure that:

- all equipment is regularly tested for condition and serviceability (e.g. stretchers and treatment tables)

- faulty equipment is marked clearly as 'NOT FOR USE' or discarded immediately
- use-by dates of consumables are routinely checked and out-of-date stock discarded
- the packaging of stock is regularly checked for intact seals and sterility
- equipment is stored safely and appropriately considering its weight (e.g. heavy equipment is stored closer to the ground)
- equipment and consumables are stored appropriately according to their frequency of use (e.g. protective gloves should be readily visible and accessible)
- infectious material is discarded according to biohazard regulations.

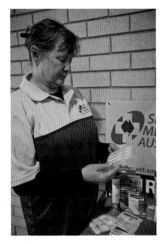

Figure 1.5 Regular equipment and product checks are part of the sports trainer's role

Relationships with other health care professionals

As a sports trainer, developing and maintaining relationships with other health care professionals is a vital part of your role in the management of athletes that you are assisting. Close liaison with health professionals is also a valuable opportunity to enhance your own continuing education.

Although sports trainers are often the first person in the sports medicine team to respond to a sports-related injury or illness, the sports trainer's role is limited according to their scope of practice and skills. Sports trainers, therefore, need to have a clear understanding of their role as a member of the sports medicine team including, in particular, the need to refer athletes to more qualified health care professionals where this is appropriate. Sports trainers must also remember that it is inappropriate and unethical for them to attempt to provide a diagnosis for any injury or health condition. A diagnosis can only be established by a health professional.

Flow chart 1.1 outlines the role of the sports trainer from the time of injury to the time when the athlete is cleared to return to play.

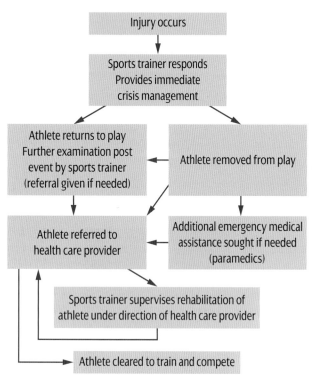

Flow chart 1.1 The sports trainer's role from injury to return to play

As can be seen from the flow chart, the sports trainer plays a role in athlete injury management, both at the early stages of management and in the course of assisting with the rehabilitation process as directed by health care professionals in the period prior to the athlete returning to play.

The following categories of health care professionals commonly form part of the sports medicine team that the sports trainer may be working or communicating with:

- doctors
- physiotherapists
- exercise and sport scientists
- psychologists
- dietitians
- podiatrists.

These health professionals may prescribe or suggest treatments or programs to the athlete, and the sports trainer may be able to assist with implementing or supervising them. For this reason, it is useful for the sports trainer to have a basic understanding of medical terminology and protocols, although the health professional will usually specify exactly what should be done and when. Ensuring that the athlete complies fully with any professional advice is an important and valuable role of the sports trainer.

The sports trainer and professionalism

Athletes, officials and health care professionals will judge a sports trainer by the following attributes.

Professional conduct

Sports trainers should work within the parameters of the Sports Trainer Code of Ethics (discussed later in this chapter) and never operate outside of their scope of practice. Always display an 'athlete first' philosophy and make the athlete's health, safety and wellbeing the first priority.

Dress and presentation

Ensure your dress and presentation are of a high standard and maintain the highest standard of personal hygiene and personal health. The dress, presentation and conduct of sports trainers all reinforce their ability to perform their duties.

Clothing should be neat, appropriate to the conditions and comply with any standards or regulations relevant to the particular sport or event. Ideally, the uniform should be sufficiently visible and recognisable so that the sports trainer can be easily identified, especially in the event of an emergency. For sports that do not specify or require a particular uniform, SMA accredited sports trainers are entitled and encouraged to wear the SMA approved uniform with the SMA logo.

Communication skills

All forms of documentation should be thorough, legible and able to be understood by the athlete and other health care professionals. Verbal communication should be clear, concise and non-threatening. When responding to an emergency or other incident, a sports trainer's capacity to remain calm and communicate clearly will assist the athlete in distress and improve the sports trainer's ability to make and implement decisions effectively.

Hand signals and other non-verbal communication

It is important to know how to communicate non-verbally with other medical staff during emergencies. This is particularly important in situations where noise or distance prevents verbal communication. To achieve effective communication in these circumstances, sports trainers and other health professionals may use a variety of hand signals to signal their intentions or request additional assistance.

It is important to remember that hand signals are not necessarily the same in all sports or even among all clubs, so the sports trainer must ensure that any hand signals to be used are understood by those to whom they are directed. Examples of hand signals that may be used are shown in Figures 1.6 to 1.12.

ASSISTANCE REQUIRED

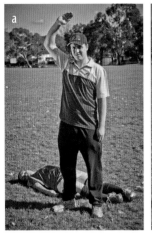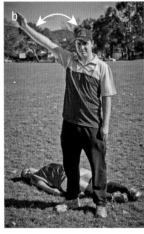

Figure 1.6 Assistance required signal – hand left (a) and right (b) over head

UNCONSCIOUS ATHLETE

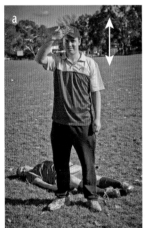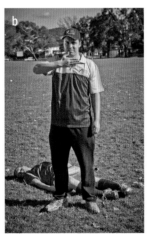

Figure 1.7 Unconscious athlete signal – hand up (a) and down (b) across face

ATHLETE NOT BREATHING

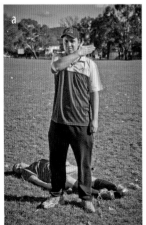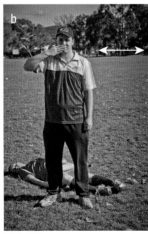

Figure 1.8 Athlete not breathing signal – hand left (a) and right (b) across mouth

SUSPECTED SPINAL INJURY

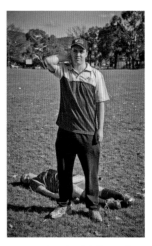

Figure 1.9 Suspected spinal injury signal

STRETCHER REQUIRED

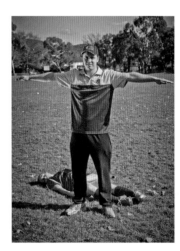

Figure 1.10 Stretcher required signal

ADDITIONAL FIRST AID SUPPLIES REQUIRED

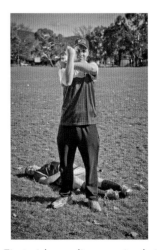

Figure 1.11 First aid supplies required signal

REMOVING AN ATHLETE FROM PLAY

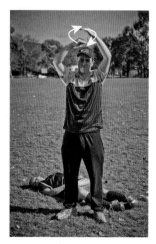

Figure 1.12 Removing an athlete from play signal – hands in circular motion above head

Sports trainer continuing education and development

Sports medicine is an ever-changing field. As new scientific and medical research is undertaken, changes in medical knowledge and practices continue to evolve and improve. These changes require that sports trainers continually seek to update their knowledge and skills in line with current standards and best practice. Continuing education also allows sports trainers to learn new techniques and further expand their skills.

Some of the continuing education options available to sports trainers are:

- SMA Level 2 Sports Trainer accreditation
- Certificate III Sports Trainer qualification
- advanced first aid and emergency care certification
- annual re-accreditation of resuscitation qualifications
- three-year re-accreditation of sports trainer and sports first aid qualifications
- SMA Safer Sport Program Short Courses
- SMA sports trainer conferences
- SMA education seminars
- The Australian Conference of Science and Medicine in Sport.

As sports trainers need to effectively manage their time to balance the differing tasks required of them and also need to communicate effectively with athletes, coaches, health professionals and others, development of both time management and communication skills is also valuable.

Sports trainer equipment

The quantity and type of equipment required for a sports trainer will be determined largely by:

- the sports trainer's designated role within the team
- specific equipment requirements of the sport
- the level of competition
- the budget.

However, a sports trainer should carry a few essential items at all times in a hip pack that contains the following items as a minimum:

- resuscitation mask
- protective gloves
- sterile gauze
- sterile gauze bandages
- triangular bandage.

The sports trainer should also have access to:

- comprehensive first aid supplies that are regularly restocked and maintained (see Appendix A for suggested minimum contents)
- ice or ice packs
- access to a telephone or mobile phone and a list of emergency telephone numbers
- notebook, documentation forms and several pens.

A copy of the latest edition of *Sports Medicine for Sports Trainers* should also be carried.

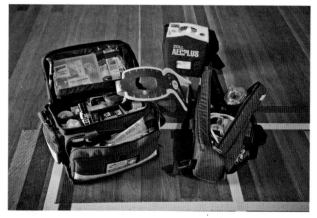

Figure 1.13 Some sports medicine supplies used by sports trainers

Documentation for sports trainers

Sports trainers must make a record of all medical encounters they have with an athlete. Correct documentation of all medical encounters provides legal protection for the sports trainer, the athlete and the sport, and can be important in the event of an insurance or compensation claim by an athlete.

In all Australian states and territories, written documentation and reporting of injuries is mandatory under workplace health and safety laws. This is especially relevant for sports trainers who are working with professional athletes as this type of legislation specifically applies to them.

All sports trainer documentation must:

- be accurate and legible
- be written in black ink, with any corrections marked and signed for
- be signed and dated by the sports trainer
- be stored in accordance with regulatory policy as determined by national or state/territory legislation and the rules or requirements of the sporting organisation or club.

An important piece of legislation relating to the collection and storage of medically related information is the *Privacy Act*. This establishes the Australian National Privacy Principles encompassing rules on the collection, use and storage of information, including medical records. Information about and explanations of the National Privacy Principles can be found on the Office of the Australian Information Commissioner website (www.privacy.gov.au).

Injury report form

It is important for the sports trainer to keep clear and accurate records of all sports-related injuries and medical conditions being managed, whether emergencies or minor incidents, regardless of how serious a sports trainer perceives the incident to be at the time.

WHY USE AN INJURY REPORT FORM?

Injury report forms provide a record of the sports trainer's observations, assessment and management of a particular injury. Injury report forms are for:

- the sports trainer's records
- the club's records
- the provision of referral information to health care professionals
- legal purposes – accurate and complete records are essential should legal action be taken against the sports trainer or the club.

SMA injury report forms also ensure that key steps in the appropriate management regimen of injured athletes are not accidently omitted, as well as providing a national standard of care to which all SMA accredited sports trainers are expected to conform.

Injury report forms are also an important part of sports injury prevention as they can be used to identify injury trends or patterns within teams, clubs or sports that can help to identify likely contributory factors. Correcting these contributory factors can reduce the likely incidence of future injuries. Injury report forms are available on the SMA website (www.sma.org.au). There is also an injury report form in Appendix C.

Athlete medical profile forms

It is important for the sports trainer to have an accurate medical profile form on file for every athlete that is completed during the pre-season and updated at least yearly. It should include information about current and previous medical conditions and injuries.

WHY USE A MEDICAL PROFILE FORM?

Medical profile forms (see Appendix D) allow the sports trainer to be aware of any specific conditions an athlete has and to thereby be prepared should an emergency arise. The forms also ensure the sports trainer has emergency contact details for every athlete under their care.

Any information gathered by the sports trainer regarding an athlete, including their medical history or injuries, is privileged information. This information must be used with discretion and must preserve the privacy and rights of the athlete as well as meeting the needs of the club. In accordance with the National Privacy Principles, the athlete must always be told why the information is being collected and that they have the right to access that information. Any data collected must be protected from misuse and loss, and from unauthorised modification.

Occasionally, the sports trainer may experience a conflict of interest, such as if they are asked to reveal information to the employing club, coach or other official about an injury or illness and its effect on the athlete's ability to compete. The sports trainer must have the athlete's permission before revealing any such information to a third party.

Equity issues in sport

A sports trainer is required to provide and promote an equitable competition environment within their sporting team/event. An understanding of harassment, discrimination and child abuse is expected of sports trainers so they may understand the detrimental effect these issues have on athlete health and wellbeing.

Harassment consists of offensive, abusive, belittling or threatening behaviour directed at a person or persons. To qualify as harassment, the behaviour must be unwelcome and the sort of behaviour a reasonable person would recognise as unwelcome.

Discrimination involves making choices about how we treat other people. Those choices can be made using real and relevant information or they can be based on prejudice, stereotypes and bias. Some discrimination, such as sexual harassment and racial discrimination, is unlawful. Other discrimination is not unlawful but it may still be unwelcome or inappropriate, such as when a coach shows favouritism towards their own child over other players. All such discrimination is undesirable if it leads to unfair treatment of players, members and other participants in recreation and sport.

What is fair discrimination?

Fair discrimination is based on actual individual differences in capability or suitability. For example, fair discrimination practices should be applied to sporting team selection. To arrive at the best possible team, coaches and selectors must discriminate between the available players to decide who will be in the starting team and what positions they will play. In junior and sub-junior sport, coaches and selectors also have an additional responsibility to ensure fair participation. Their selection choices should be based upon relevant criteria, such as ability, attitude, effort and attendance at practice, which are all fair and legitimate criteria to apply to team selection.

What is unlawful discrimination?

Equal opportunity laws require that all people should be treated equally and not discriminated against because of:

- race
- age
- gender
- religion
- marital status
- sexuality
- disability
- pregnancy.

However, some of these factors, including age, gender and whether a person has a disability, can have significant effects on sporting ability. To take these differences into account, and to ensure there is fair competition, it is allowable and appropriate for teams to be organised into groups, such as age groups or sometimes single-sex groups.

Child abuse in sport

Child abuse can occur through someone doing something harmful to a child or young person, or by not providing for or protecting a child or young person. Child abuse can cause long-lasting emotional, physical and behavioural damage.

The four main types of child abuse are set out below.

1 Sexual abuse/sexual misconduct: any sexual act or sexual threat imposed on a child or young person, including suggestive behaviour and inappropriate touching. For example, a coach holding their arms longer than necessary around a participant to teach a golf swing or tennis serve, or watching an athlete change or shower.

2 Physical abuse: non-accidental injury and/or harm to a child or young person caused by a parent, caregiver or another person, including other children. Examples include hitting or physically punishing a young person for losing an event, pushing or shoving them or throwing equipment at them.

3 Emotional abuse: includes any behaviour that may emotionally or psychologically harm a child or young person, including verbal abuse, threats, bullying, harassment or excessive and unreasonable demands. Examples include continual yelling or name-calling, belittling children verbally, racial vilification or encouraging violent behaviour at training or at the game.

4 Neglect: occurs where a child or young person is at risk of harm or is harmed by the failure to provide them with the basic physical and emotional necessities of life. In sport, neglect can include keeping a child on the field who has sustained an injury to improve the chance of winning the game or discouraging children from drinking water before a competition as it may add weight and compromise a weigh-in.

'Play by the Rules' is a partnership between the Australian Sports Commission and all state/territory sport and recreation and anti-discrimination agencies and provides further information and online learning on how to prevent and deal with discrimination, harassment and child abuse in the sport and recreation industry (see www.playbytherules.com.au).

Sports trainer code of ethics

All SMA accredited sports trainers agree to operate in accordance with the SMA Sports Trainer Code of Ethics. This code describes best practice policy for all sports trainers.

Sports trainers must agree to, and operate in accordance with, the code's three key principles:

1 It is the primary role of sports trainers to apply their knowledge and skills to help make sport and recreation safer. This is achieved by implementing appropriate injury prevention regimes; in the case of injury, it is achieved by applying appropriate initial management procedures and by referring injuries, as necessary, to a more qualified health professional for further advice and management.

2 The sports trainer must clearly understand their defined roles and responsibilities and has a moral responsibility to work within the limits of their qualifications and, hence, not assume roles outside of those predetermined ones. In keeping within the limits of their qualifications, the sports trainer must, if appropriate, refer injuries to a more qualified health professional.

3 Sports trainers are trained to provide definite skills and knowledge (as outlined in their roles and responsibilities) to sports clubs/sporting events, and it is acceptable to receive remuneration for their time and involvement with that club/event. However, it is clearly inappropriate, and outside of the role for which the sports trainer has been educated, for a sports trainer to offer themselves as a primary health care practitioner and charge on a fee-for-service basis.

If a sports trainer is found to be acting outside of the above guidelines, they will be investigated by the SMA and may have their certification/accreditation revoked.

Chapter Two

FUNCTIONAL MUSCULO-SKELETAL ANATOMY

LEARNING OUTCOMES

Use the correct anatomical terminology to:

1 Describe the major anatomical terms
2 Identify major skeletal bones of the body
3 Explain the function of different joint structures and their respective actions
4 Identify major muscles of the body
5 Explain the major types of muscle contraction

ASSESSMENT OF OUTCOMES

Underpinning knowledge

Oral or written questions may be asked, relating to the structure of the musculoskeletal system, which require the correct use of anatomical terminology. You may also be asked to complete an online task or workbook with related activities.

Practical demonstration

You may be asked to explain the relationships between different anatomical structures. You may also be asked to show the sites of possible injuries and reference them using correct anatomical terminology.

Scenario

You may be required to identify the site of injuries on an injured athlete using correct anatomical terminology.

Introduction

This chapter contains a brief introduction to the musculoskeletal system of the human body. A basic understanding of the structures of bones, joints and muscles and how they relate and interact helps sports trainers by:

- providing a basic understanding of how the musculoskeletal structures of the body function, especially in the production of movement
- allowing sports trainers to more accurately describe the location of an injury, especially for the purposes of referral
- enhancing the ability of sports trainers to recognise when an injury has caused a change to the normal appearance or function of a region of the body.

Although this chapter is limited to musculoskeletal anatomy, an understanding of other body systems, and particularly how they are affected by sport and physical activity, is also useful and is an appropriate area of continuing education for sports trainers to pursue.

Anatomical terminology

Descriptive terminology is necessary in anatomy to describe the position and relationship of different anatomical structures to each other with clarity and certainty. It is necessary to be familiar with some of this terminology to be able to accurately describe parts of the musculoskeletal system and to accurately identify sites of injury.

To allow for clear and accurate communication regarding body movement and position, there is a standard position that all terminology is related to. This is known as the 'anatomical position'. The anatomical position is standing erect and facing forwards with the arms by the sides with palms facing forward and fingers extended.

All terminology relates to this anatomical position. The terms regarding the location and relationship of body parts are shown in Table 2.1 and Figure 2.1.

Description of anatomical movements

To enable accurate communication with other health professionals, the sports trainer must be fluent in the terminology regarding movement.

The terms regarding movement are set out in Table 2.2 and Figure 2.2.

The skeletal system

On average, the skeleton of an adult consists of 206 bones. It has five functions:

1 providing the basic shape and support of the body
2 protecting internal organs
3 producing movement in conjunction with the muscles
4 storing minerals, in particular calcium and phosphorus
5 producing red blood cells in the bone marrow.

Table 2.1 Anatomical terms denoting relationship and comparison

Term	Description
TERMS OF RELATIONSHIP	
Anterior	Nearer to the front of the body (e.g. the sternum is on the anterior side of the body)
Posterior	Nearer to the back of the body (e.g. the scapula is on the posterior side of the body)
Superior	Nearer to the top of the head (e.g. the eyes are superior to the mouth)
Inferior	Nearer to the soles of the feet (e.g. the liver is inferior to the heart)
Medial	Nearer to the midline of the body (e.g. the heart is medial to the lungs)
Lateral	Away from the midline of the body (e.g. the ears are on the lateral side of the head)
TERMS OF COMPARISON	
Proximal	Nearer to the trunk (e.g. the shoulder is proximal to the hand)
Distal	Further from the trunk (e.g. the foot is distal to the hip)
Superficial	Near to the surface or on the surface (e.g. skin is superficial to muscle)
Deep	Further from the surface (e.g. the tendons are deep to the skin)
Ipsilateral	On the same side of the body (e.g. the gallbladder is ipsilateral to the liver)
Contralateral	On the opposite side of the body (e.g. the spleen is contralateral to the liver)

Anterior
Towards the front
e.g. The sternum is on the anterior side of the body

Posterior
Towards the back
e.g. The scapula is on the posterior side of the body

Superior
Towards the head or upper part of the structure
e.g. The eyes are superior to the mouth

Inferior
Towards the back
e.g. The liver is inferior to the heart

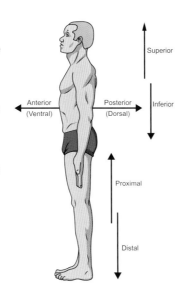

Proximal
Closer to the trunk than something else on the limb
e.g. The shoulder is proximal to the hand

Distal
Further from the trunk than something else on the limb
e.g. The foot is distal to the hip

Medial
Towards the midline of the body
e.g. The heart is medial to the lungs

Lateral
Away from the midline of the body
e.g. The ears are on the lateral side of the body

Superficial
Towards or close to the surface of the body
e.g. The skin is superficial to muscle

Deep
Away from the surface of the body
e.g. The tendons are deep to the skin

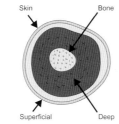

Figure 2.1 The anatomical position and terms of location

Structure of bone

Bone is a living tissue that is constantly undergoing remodelling in response to the stress placed on it. Bones have an outer, compact and dense layer and an inner, spongy centre. This structure gives bones strength and rigidity but at a light weight. Blood cells are formed by the bone marrow in the spongy centre of the bone.

Table 2.2 Terms describing movement

Term	Description
Flexion	Movement at a joint resulting in a decrease in the angle between the two bones
Extension	Movement at a joint resulting in an increase in the angle between the two bones
Abduction	Movement away from the midline of the body
Adduction	Movement towards the midline of the body
Inversion	Movement of the sole of the foot inwards
Eversion	Movement of the sole of the foot outwards
Plantar flexion	Pointing the foot
Dorsiflexion	Lifting the foot towards the shin
Rotation	Rotation of a bone around its own axis
Internal rotation	Rotation of the bone towards the midline of the body
External rotation	Rotation of the bone away from the midline of the body
Circumduction	The distal end of the bone follows a circular path and the proximal end stays stable. Circumduction is a combination of flexion, abduction, extension and adduction
Supination	Outward rotation of the forearm (palm faces anterior)
Pronation	Inward rotation of the forearm (palm faces posterior)
Elevation	Raising the shoulder towards the head
Depression	Lowering of the shoulder towards the feet

The contact or 'articular' surfaces of bones within joints are usually covered with hard, smooth cartilage that provides for smooth movement of the joints.

Bones are generally classified according to their shape:

- long bones (e.g. the femur)
- short bones (e.g. the carpal bones of the wrist)
- flat bones (e.g. the ribs)
- irregular bones (e.g. the vertebrae).

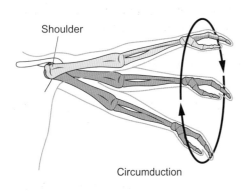

(a) Circumduction

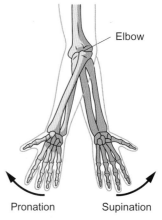

(b) Pronation/supination

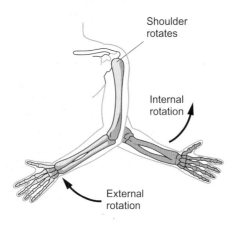

(c) External/interal rotation

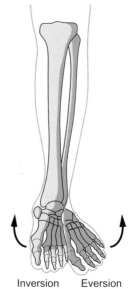

(d) Inversion/eversion

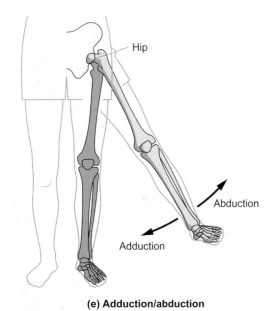

(e) Adduction/abduction

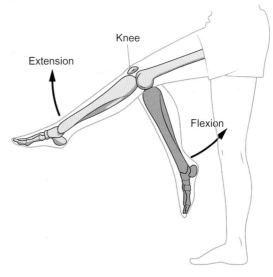

(f) Extension/flexion

Figure 2.2 Anatomical movement direction terms

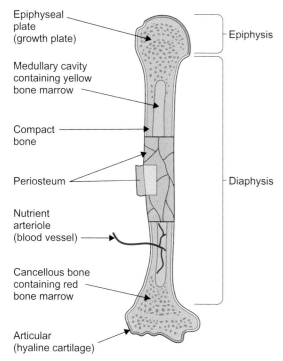

Figure 2.3 Structure of bone

THE MAJOR BONES OF THE SKELETON

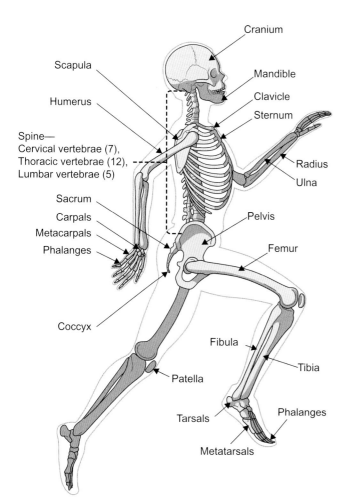

Figure 2.4 Major bones of the skeleton

INJURIES TO BONE

The most common injuries to bone include:

- acute fractures as a result of direct or indirect trauma
- stress fractures as a result of overuse
- bruising (bleeding in the bone)
- damage to the bone growth plate (epiphysis) in children or adolescents.

Joints

A joint is the meeting point between bones. It will usually allow for a controlled movement between the adjoining bones that is produced by the contraction of muscles attached to both bones.

Classification of joints

There are several different types of joints within the body that allow different types and amounts of movement. Some joints need to be very stable whereas others need to be very mobile. Joints are usually classified according to their structure (synovial, cartilaginous or fibrous), but can be further classified according to the amount of mobility they allow or according to their shape, as outlined in the descriptions below. Joints that allow more movement are usually most prone to injury.

SADDLE JOINT

Saddle joints have two combined concave/convex surfaces that mostly allow movement in two directions. The joint at the base of the thumb (the first carpometacarpal joint) is a saddle joint.

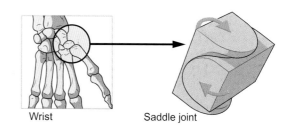

Figure 2.5 Saddle joint

HINGE JOINT

Hinge joints allow movement in one direction only. For example, the elbow is a hinge joint that allows extension and flexion.

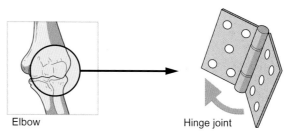

Figure 2.6 Hinge joint

PLANE JOINT

Plane joints have relatively flat surfaces that permit the bones to slide on each other and usually allow only a small range of movement. An example is the acromioclavicular joint between the scapula and clavicle.

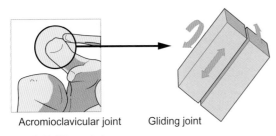

Acromioclavicular joint   Gliding joint

Figure 2.7 Plane joint

ELLIPSOID JOINT

Ellipsoid joints are similar to ball and socket joints but only allow movement in two directions.

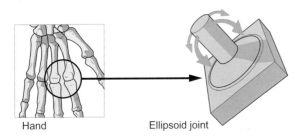

Hand   Ellipsoid joint

Figure 2.8 Ellipsoid joint

BALL-AND-SOCKET JOINT

These joints consist of a cup-shaped socket with a matching ball that allows movement in all directions. The amount of movement is affected by the tightness of the fit between the two surfaces. For example, the shoulder is a highly mobile ball-and-socket joint, whereas the hip is a less mobile ball-and-socket joint.

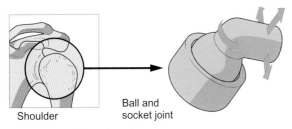

Shoulder   Ball and socket joint

Figure 2.9 Ball-and-socket joint

CONDYLOID JOINT

These joints only allow active movement in two directions but can also allow passive movement in a third axis of direction. For example, the metacarpophalangeal joints between the hand and the fingers.

PIVOT JOINT

Pivot joints allow movement around a single axis, usually rotation. Examples are the articulation between the first two cervical vertebrae or the superior radioulnar joint of the elbow.

Structure of joints

Most joints contain the structures outlined in Table 2.3.

Injuries to joints

The most common injuries to joints include:

- dislocation
- subluxation (incomplete or partial dislocation)
- fracture of bone associated with the joint
- damage to soft tissue structures in and around the joint, such as ligament tears or ruptures.

Ligaments

Ligaments are fibrous bands of connective tissue that attach two or more bones together at a joint. They enhance stability at the joint by maintaining the alignment of the bones and limiting the range of movement at the joint. In synovial joints ligaments also help to enclose the joint and retain synovial fluid.

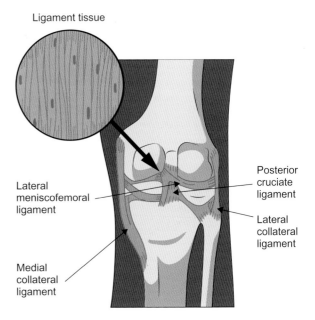

Ligament tissue

Lateral meniscofemoral ligament

Posterior cruciate ligament

Lateral collateral ligament

Medial collateral ligament

Posterior view of the knee joint

Figure 2.10 Ligaments of the knee

Table 2.3 Joint structures

Structure	Description	Function
Bone	The hard tissue that forms the strong internal framework of the body	• Provides support and protection • The shape of the bones may limit the range of movement at the joint
Cartilage	The smooth lining on the ends of the bones in a joint	• Protects the ends of the bones from wear and tear • Reduces friction
Joint cavity	The space between the articulating bones at a joint, containing synovial fluid	• Provides space for the movement of bones to occur
Joint capsule	A fibrous sleeve surrounding and enclosing the joint	• Defines the joint cavity • Holds the fluid in the joint
Synovial membrane	Thin lining on the inside of the joint capsule	• Produces synovial fluid
Synovial fluid	The thick fluid found in a synovial joint	• Lubricates the joint for smooth movement • Provides nourishment for the lining cartilage • Keeps the lining cartilages from touching each other
Ligaments	Strong, fibrous inelastic bands connecting bone to bone. Ligaments may be either outside or part of the joint capsule. Ligaments are closely related to the joint capsule	• Help hold the joint together • Give stability to the joint • Help limit the range of motion at the joint

Injuries to ligaments

The most common injuries to ligaments occur as a result of overstretching, which leads to tearing of the ligament tissue. Damage can range from tearing of several fibres to a complete rupture.

The muscular system

Muscles are contractile tissues that can produce movement in the body. Muscles comprise 25–45% of our total body weight. There are over 650 skeletal muscles controlled by the body's nervous system.

There are three types of muscles in the body. They are:

1 skeletal muscle (under voluntary control)
2 cardiac muscle (found only in the heart and under automatic body control)
3 smooth muscle (found in various organs and under automatic body control).

This book focuses on skeletal muscle as it is the most prevalent muscle type, as well as being the most susceptible to sporting injuries.

Function of skeletal muscle

The function of skeletal muscle is to produce movement of the bones of the skeleton by either:

■ shortening when the muscle contracts, which pulls the bones to which the muscle is attached closer together
■ lengthening when the muscle relaxes, allowing the bones to move further apart.

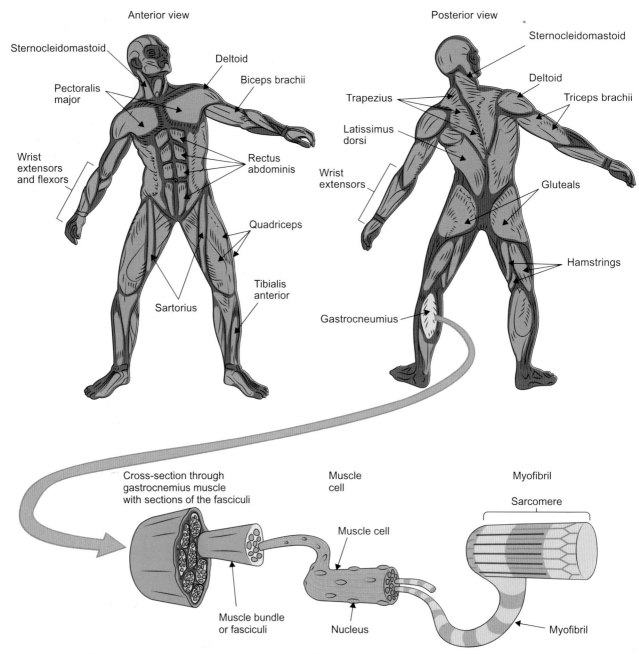

Figure 2.11 Skeletal muscle: major muscles of the body and structure

Structure of skeletal muscle

Most muscles join one bone to another and usually have one or more attachments on relatively less mobile bone or bones called the *origin*, and an attachment on the bone that is moved called the *insertion*. The insertion is usually relatively more distal to the origin.

The main body of the muscle is called the *belly*. It contains many large bundles of parallel muscle fibres, each of which are made of many individual muscle fibres. Muscle fibres are comprised of proteins and connective tissue that contract and shorten upon stimulation by a nerve. Skeletal muscles have an extensive blood supply to provide the muscle with oxygen and nutrients to produce energy for movement and to remove waste products.

Muscles are often attached to bone by *tendons*, but some are attached directly by other types of connective tissue. Tendons are slightly elastic tissues that cannot actively contract but transfer the contractile force of the muscle to the bones they are attached to.

There are many different shapes and types of skeletal muscles, with varying arrangements of muscle bellies, tendons and attachments to bones.

Muscle contraction

The primary action of skeletal muscles is to produce or control movement.

Active shortening of a muscle is known as a *concentric* contraction. Concentric contractions occur when nerve stimulation causes the muscle fibres to contract and shorten the overall length of the muscle, thereby pulling on the bone to which it is attached. An example is the biceps muscle that pulls the forearm towards the shoulder.

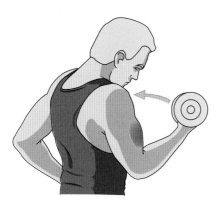

Concentric contraction

Figure 2.12 Concentric contraction

Muscles can also undergo an *eccentric* contraction. This is when the muscle is stimulated to contract while the muscle is lengthening, usually to control the rate or direction of movement of the limb. For example, the biceps in the upper arm contracts eccentrically when lowering a weight held in the hand.

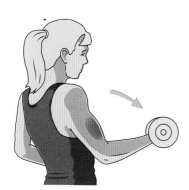

Eccentric contraction

Figure 2.13 Eccentric contraction

Muscle can also contract without changing the overall muscle length, such as when a muscle contracts against an immovable force. This is known as an *isometric* contraction.

Injuries to skeletal muscle

The most common injuries to skeletal muscle include:
- strain – overstretching or tearing of the muscle fibres. Strains may range from a few fibres to an almost complete tear.
- bruising – bleeding in the muscle. Also known as a contusion or haematoma

- rupture – a complete tear through the muscle
- avulsion – separation of the muscle attachment from the bone.

Tendons

Tendons are tough, inelastic but flexible bands of connective tissue that attach muscle to bone. Some tendons are surrounded by tendon sheaths that are filled with synovial fluid to minimise friction and facilitate movement. They have a limited blood supply, which can make them difficult to repair if injured.

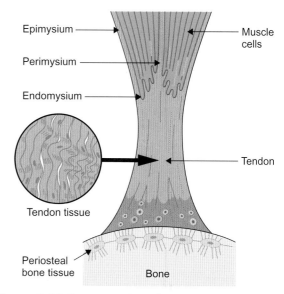

Figure 2.14 Structure of tendon

Function of tendons
The primary functions of tendons are to:
- connect muscle to bone
- facilitate movement.

Common injuries to tendons
The most common injuries to tendons include:
- strain – overstretching or tearing of the tendon fibres
- tendinopathy – overuse or degenerative injuries of the tendon
- rupture – a complete tear of the tendon.

Bursae

Bursae are small sacs of fibrous tissue filled with synovial fluid. Bursae are normally located around joints and in places where ligaments and tendons pass over bone or other anatomical structures. They may, however, be formed in other places in response to unusual friction or pressure.

The primary function of a bursa is to reduce friction between the structures they separate.

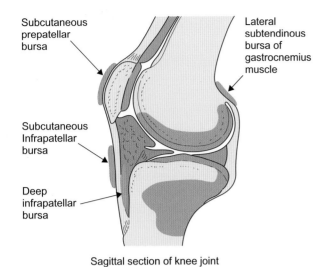

Sagittal section of knee joint

Figure 2.15 Bursa of the knee

Common injuries to bursae

The most common injury to bursae is inflammation, which is sometimes referred to as bursitis. Bursitis can occur as a result of gradual overuse or from direct trauma.

Chapter Three

PREVENTING SPORTS INJURIES

LEARNING OUTCOMES

Improve safety in sport by identifying and reducing risks to players' safety, in particular by conducting safe and appropriate warm-up and training sessions, which are an important part of the role of a sports trainer.

1 Explain the role of a warm-up.
2 Explain the preferred timing and duration of a warm-up.
3 Demonstrate a range of warm-up exercises appropriate for a variety of sports.
4 Explain the role of a cool-down.
5 Explain the preferred timing and duration of a cool-down.
6 Demonstrate a range of cool-down activities appropriate for a variety of sports.
7 Recognise precautions for warm-ups, cool-downs and stretching activities.
8 Demonstrate safe stretching activities.
9 Identify a range of sporting protective equipment.
10 Demonstrate the use of various sporting protective equipment.

ASSESSMENT OF OUTCOMES

Underpinning knowledge

Oral or written questions may be asked relating to the conduct of safe warm-up, stretching and cool-down programs. You may also be asked to complete an online task or workbook with related activities.

Practical demonstration

You may be asked to instruct or demonstrate to your peers a comprehensive warm-up, stretching and cool-down program.

Scenario

You may be asked to give an information session to athletes about the necessity of a comprehensive warm-up, stretching and cool-down program.

Introduction

Sports injury prevention is an important part of risk management in sport. Although sport and physical activities have many benefits, especially improved health and wellbeing, there is also an ongoing associated risk that participants may sustain an injury while participating in sport or training. Sporting clubs should therefore have in place a coordinated approach to sports injury prevention and injury management by having available properly trained sports medicine personnel, equipment and clearly understood procedures. Athlete health and wellbeing must always remain the primary consideration over all others in sport.

The risk of injury in sport can be significantly reduced by identifying and limiting or removing known risk factors. A systematic approach to sports injury prevention has been proven to greatly reduce the number and severity of sports injuries when scientifically based approaches and techniques are used. These techniques can often be implemented effectively by sports teams of all levels, generally at low cost, as they do not require much equipment or any special equipment.

Sports trainers have an important risk management role within sporting organisations and clubs in identifying and correcting risk factors to which their athletes may be exposed, as well as being properly prepared to respond to adverse incidents that may occur. They can assist in sports injury prevention in many ways, including ensuring the safety of grounds and equipment, and especially assisting with player preparation by designing or supervising warm-up and injury prevention exercise programs appropriate to the sport. Sports trainers can also assist player preparation and injury prevention with preventative taping and by ensuring other protective equipment is well chosen and properly fitted, taking into account the specific needs of the athlete and the demands of the sport.

General injury prevention principles

Sports Medicine Australia (SMA) advises adopting the following general injury prevention principles:

1   Ensure playing facilities and equipment are well maintained and risk free.

2   Ensure athletes always warm up before training and competition.

3   Ensure athletes achieve as high a level of fitness as possible, including strength, coordination, flexibility and endurance, as well as speed, power and agility appropriate to the sport.

4   Develop athlete skills and techniques appropriate to the chosen sport.

5   Ensure athletes wear appropriate protective equipment.

6   Ensure athletes obey the rules of the sport and respect the safety of team mates and opponents.

7   Encourage balanced competition.

8   Maximise recovery with appropriate rest, nutrition, cool-downs etc, before athletes resume training or playing again.

9   Ensure full recovery from injuries before allowing an athlete to return to sport.

All of these points of general injury prevention are important in reducing the incidence of injury to athletes.

Sports injury surveillance

Sports injury surveillance is the collection of information related to sports injuries. As mentioned in Chapter 1, sports trainers can improve sports injury prevention programs by collecting information about how, when and where injuries occurred. This information can be used to identify patterns or groups of injuries that may have a common cause that can, in turn, be remedied. Injury surveillance starts with the collection of information on a suitable injury report form. This can be either a paper based system or an online system such as Sports Injury Tracker (see www.sportsinjurytracker.com.au).

Medical emergency planning

As part of their risk management processes sports clubs should have well-developed medical emergency prevention and management systems in place. A sporting organisation's medical emergency plan should be summarised in a written document that is available to and clearly understood by all people within the organisation so that, in the event of a medical incident, whether major or minor, everyone knows what to do and what their particular role is at that time. To be effective, training should also be carried out within the club or team using simulated emergencies to ensure that the plan can be implemented effectively.

The Sports Medicine Australia SmartPlay program has developed a planning guide called 'Medical emergency planning: a practical guide for clubs' that is available on the SmartPlay website (www.smartplay.com.au). It has a checklist and action plan template that can be used to develop a medical emergency plan.

Extrinsic and intrinsic risk factors for injury

Risk factors for injury are often described as being either extrinsic, in other words external to the player, or intrinsic, which are internal factors. For example, extrinsic risk factors include the playing environment or sports equipment such as bats or balls that could cause an injury. Intrinsic risk factors include the player's age, skill level, fitness and other factors affecting their suitability for a specific sport or sporting task, including biomechanical factors such as leg length differences or muscle weakness or imbalance.

The sporting environment

The sports trainer's role includes checking that the playing environment is as safe as it possibly can be. This could involve minimising tripping or falling hazards, such as holes in the playing surface, sprinklers, unsecured floor matting etc, or checking that goal post padding is in place and properly secured.

The hardness of sporting grounds and certain types of grass or surface covering can also influence the incidence, type and severity of sports injuries. Ground hardness is considered to be a risk factor especially for lower limb overuse injury as well as skin injuries, bruises and other contact-related injuries. Surface traction can be a factor with different types of grass or artificial surfaces, especially in non-contact lower limb injuries, due to the shoe either slipping along or excessively binding with the surface. The types of grass and hardness of grounds can vary significantly between regions and may depend largely on prevailing weather patterns, soil types etc. Gaining extra knowledge about these types of risk factors is useful to sports trainers as they are then able to advise sporting clubs or event organisers as to the suitability of the playing surface.

The weather is another environmental risk factor for sports injury or illness. Excessively hot or cold weather can negatively affect a player's coordination, which can lead to an increased risk of injury as well as to medical conditions such as hyperthermia or hypothermia (discussed further in Chapter 7). To ensure players' health and wellbeing is properly protected, another important role for sports trainers is checking that they are properly hydrated and have suitable clothing for the prevailing weather conditions.

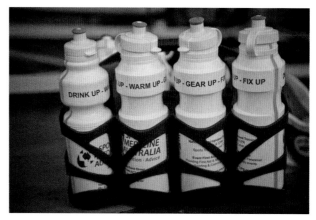

Figure 3.1 Sports injury prevention involves several components

Warm-up and injury prevention programs

Warm-up programs help to prepare athletes for sport both physically and mentally. They help to reduce injuries as well as improve sporting performance. A properly designed warm-up is essential for both training sessions and competition, although the type of warm-up program used might be very different. Warm-up and training programs will also vary depending on the specific sport as well as on factors such as the age and skill level of the participants.

Although warm-up programs help to reduce injuries in their own right, warm-ups can be combined with specific injury prevention programs, especially at training sessions. Injury prevention programs usually concentrate on improving strength, balance and coordination, which reduce the athlete's risk of being injured while training or playing.

To be effective in reducing injuries and improving performance it is essential that there is a high level of compliance with the program. To improve athlete compliance, the coach and other officials should support the program and those responsible for delivering it to the athletes. It is also helpful if the athletes have a clear understanding of the reasons for the program and the anticipated benefits it will provide.

Warm-up

Warm-up prepares the athlete for training and competition. Warm-up exercises are designed, amongst other things, to:

- increase blood flow to the exercising muscles
- improve muscle contractions and, therefore, force production
- reduce muscle tightness to increase flexibility
- decrease stiffness of joints and connective tissue such as tendons

- increase the sensitivity and conduction speed of nerve endings and nerves, which can then improve coordination and reaction time
- prepare the heart and lungs to improve the delivery of oxygen to the body
- mentally prepare the athlete for the upcoming event.

These factors all lead to a decreased chance of injury as well as improved sporting performance.

PLANNING A WARM-UP – GENERAL PRINCIPLES AND OTHER CONSIDERATIONS

In planning warm-up and other training programs, a useful set of principles to keep in mind is sometimes referred to as the 'SPIED' factors.

- **Specificity** of the exercise – the warm-up activity should include the specific muscles and movements to be used in the subsequent activity.
- **Participant's** energy levels – it is important to conserve the athlete's energy for the event to follow.
- **Intensity** of the exercise – the warm-up should be sufficiently intense to gently increase body temperature. A good guide is that participants should be able to talk with their exercise partners for the duration of the session.
- **Environmental** conditions – in cool or cold conditions, the duration of the warm-up will usually need to be longer whereas, in warm or hot conditions, a long or intense warm-up could decrease performance by exhausting the players.
- **Duration** of the exercise – the duration of the warm-up will take into consideration the time available and how long it is before the event starts, as well as the environmental and energy level factors mentioned above.

COMPONENTS OF THE WARM-UP

Warm-up activities should include all major muscle groups and involve moving the joints through their normal range of motion for that sport. Ideally, warm-up activities should also be interesting or fun to perform so the participants are properly engaged and concentrating on performing them properly.

The actual components of the warm-up or training program can vary considerably, but a structure that has been found to be useful in reducing injuries and improving performance, especially for sports that involve running and jumping activities, consists of the following elements:

1 Running drills or other low intensity activities that gradually increase circulation to increase muscle and body temperature. Especially for sports that involve running, these drills can gradually progress from walking or light jogging to include more complex and higher demand movements such as running with knee lifts, shuttle runs, carioca running and many others, preferably those specific to the nature of the sport. More advanced and complex running drills can increase running speed and improve technique as well as increase muscle flexibility and circulation (see Figure 3.2). Additional suitable warm-up activities include swimming, rowing, cycling or other activities that are specific to the actual sport.

2 Strengthening exercises for the major muscle groups used in the particular sport. Properly constructed exercise programs for sports injury prevention and performance take into consideration the way muscles work together in producing sporting movements. The goal is to improve controlled muscle power throughout the full range of movement and to develop muscle balance rather than just developing raw power or the size of individual muscles (see Figures 3.3 and 3.4).

3 Balance and body control exercises. These are designed to improve balance and coordination and to correct the alignment of the body segments during sporting movements, which in turn improves the athlete's ability to avoid situations where an injury is likely to occur. For example, research has shown a significant reduction in the number of lower joint injuries such as ankle sprains in athletes who have

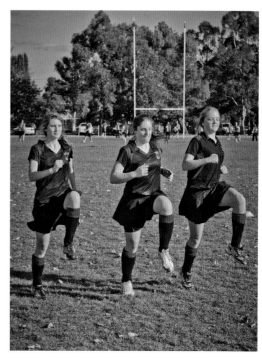

Figure 3.2 Running drills are often included in warm-up programs

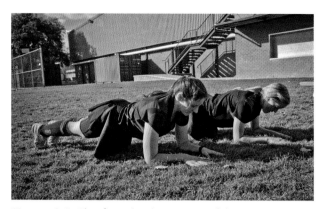

Figure 3.3 The front bridge is a useful core strengthening exercise

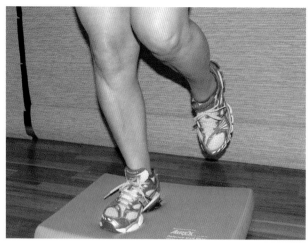

Figure 3.5 Body control exercises on a balance mat

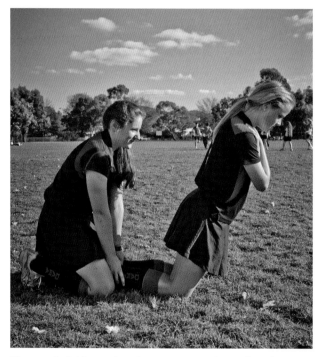

Figure 3.4 Hamstring lowers can reduce the chance of hamstring strains

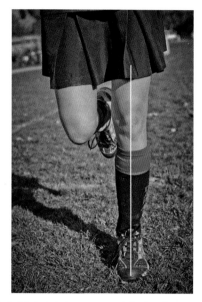

Figure 3.6 Maintaining correct limb alignment is important

undertaken programs with exercises designed to improve their balance. These exercises often incorporate an unstable surface, such as a wobble board or balance mat, but can also be done effectively on any playing surface (see Figure 3.5). Ensuring that correct lower limb alignment is properly maintained during movements is an important component of body control exercises (see Figure 3.6). Balance and body control exercises can also incorporate sports-related tasks and can be performed in pairs or larger groups (see Figure 3.7).

4 Sports specific exercises. Warm-up and training programs usually progress towards increasingly sports specific exercises that simulate part or all of a sports specific task

and gradually increase the range of movement and speed to enhance flexibility and readiness for sport. This is sometimes referred to as a dynamic warm-up (see Figure 3.8). For example, after warming up a footballer will practise kicking with gradually increasing force or intensity. To be effective as a training or injury prevention strategy these exercises should be performed in a controlled way with proper technique, control and limb alignment throughout the activity. Practising jumping, landing and side-stepping or cutting techniques is also particularly important for sports that incorporate these movements (see Figure 3.9). Pre-participation warm-ups often finish with a specific game-related activity where participants perform movements that are similar to or identical to those to be used in the actual game or training session (see Figure 3.10).

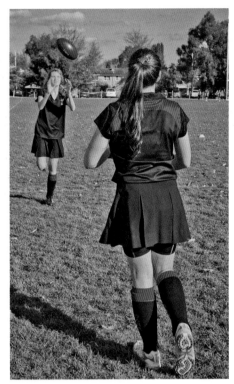

Figure 3.7 Balance exercises improve coordination and skills

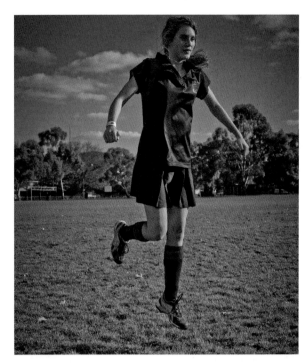

Figure 3.9 Training to improve a safe landing technique

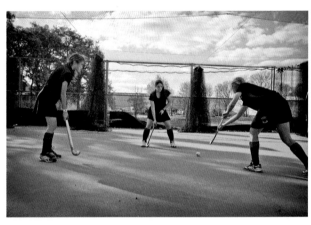

Figure 3.10 Practising sports specific skills

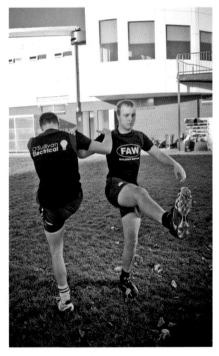

Figure 3.8 Dynamic warm-up exercises

Maintaining flexibility and keeping warm during an event

To maintain the benefits of the warm-up activities, players need to keep moving and to keep warm during inactive periods. This is particularly relevant for reserves or interchange players. Muscle temperature falls quickly after exercise stops so it is important to move from the warm-up into the main

activity as soon as possible. To decrease heat loss tracksuits or warm clothing should be worn during periods of inactivity, especially in cold conditions; alternatively, gentle movements such as walking, light jogging or cycling should be continued until taking the field of play.

Injury prevention programs

Injury prevention programs used especially at training sessions are often structured similarly to warm-up programs, but they usually have a greater emphasis on improving strength, coordination and sports specific skills. They are also usually conducted at a higher intensity than the warm-up programs used immediately before competition and have a high degree of emphasis on improving balance and coordination. Because these programs concentrate on developing the athlete's strength as well as control of movement by the nervous system, they are sometimes referred to as neuromuscular training programs.

Injury prevention programs often include improving techniques in sport specific skills such as jumping, landing, sidestepping and other sports tasks where injuries often occur. In addition to reducing the likelihood of injury, injury prevention programs usually have the added advantage of improving the athlete's sporting performance. Evidence from research has shown that properly constructed injury prevention programs are highly effective in reducing sports injuries, especially lower limb musculoskeletal injuries. Well-designed injury prevention programs can also include endurance, strength and conditioning training components to maximise the effectiveness of the training time. Exercise scientists and physiotherapists can assist with advice on suitable conditioning and injury prevention programs.

Stretching and flexibility

Flexibility is important in many sports. Stretching can increase flexibility and the range of movement available at a joint by both increasing the length of muscles and decreasing stiffness in connective tissue such as tendons. There are a number of different specific techniques for stretching and increasing the range of movement that can be included as part of an athlete's training program. These might be particularly relevant for athletes competing in sports where a high degree of flexibility is important. Stretching can also reduce muscle tension, increase circulation and make the body feel more relaxed.

However, research has shown that muscle stretching can also temporarily decrease muscle power, which means that stretching to increase muscle length should not usually be done immediately before sport. Although static stretches have been demonstrated to increase overall range of movement when performed correctly and regularly, research has found that they can reduce muscle power for a period of time. For example, static calf stretches can decrease vertical jump height for up to 45 minutes. Dynamic stretches have also been found to temporarily decrease muscle power, but not by as much as static stretches. Warm-ups and exercises that involve a full range of movement can also gradually increase flexibility, and these can be done immediately before sport or exercise. For athletes who require flexibility in their sport or who have a limited range of movement, a stretching program is recommended; however, stretching should take place after either training or competition or several hours before hand.

When and how to stretch

Stretching refers to activities that lengthen the muscle and the associated tendon and other connective tissue. It involves positioning the body in such a way that the muscle to be stretched is elongated as much as possible. With a sound knowledge of anatomy, stretches can be designed that target either isolated muscles or groups of muscles. Recent research suggests that, to achieve useful and lasting increases in muscle length, a greater volume of stretching is required than was previously thought to be the case.

To stretch safely and effectively:

- warm up prior to stretching
- stretch to the point of the onset of strain, not pain
- stretch gently and slowly – do not stretch quickly or bounce
- remain relaxed and do not hold your breath
- hold stretches for a minimum of 20 seconds
- perform each stretch at least 3 times on at least 4 days per week
- use a variety of stretches for each muscle group, especially for muscles that cross more than one joint (for example, the hamstring group of the thigh)
- do not stretch immediately before competition or training.

Types of stretching used in sport

There are three main types of stretching commonly used in sport for injury prevention and performance improvement:

1 static stretching
2 dynamic stretching
3 proprioceptive neuromuscular facilitation (PNF) stretching.

Due to the different effects these are thought to achieve, a stretching program will often include some or all of these types of stretching.

STATIC STRETCHING

Static stretching involves an athlete adopting a position of near maximum stretch for the targeted muscle and holding that position for a prolonged period. Scientific research suggests that static stretching is the most effective type of stretching for increasing muscle length but is not as effective as dynamic stretching for decreasing tendon stiffness. Static stretching has also been found to temporarily decrease muscle power, probably due to protective muscle reflexes being triggered by the stretch.

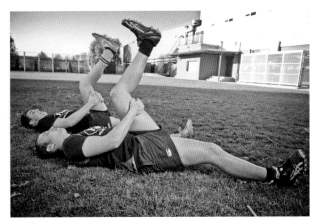

Figure 3.11 Static stretching to increase hamstring muscle length

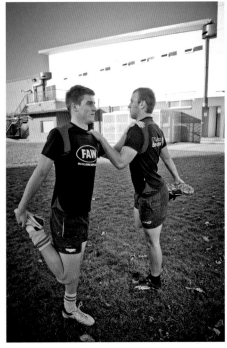

Figure 3.12 Static stretching to increase quadricep muscle length

DYNAMIC STRETCHES

Dynamic stretches, also known as active stretches, are movements that take the joints through the full range of motion, causing the muscles to be stretched dynamically. To avoid tearing or overstretching of the muscles, these stretches should only be performed after warming up properly. Dynamic stretches are often based on the specific movements involved in the sport. They have been found to be more effective for reducing tendon stiffness, but they are not as effective for increasing muscle length as static stretches.

PNF STRETCHES

Proprioceptive neuromuscular facilitation (PNF) stretching involves adopting a position of maximum stretch of a muscle and then contracting the stretched muscle against resistance. Contracting

the stretched muscle is thought to cause a temporary fatigue effect that reduces its resistance to stretch once the muscle is relaxed, which then allows the athlete to move to a position of increased muscle length. A partner can be used to provide the resistance for the stretched muscle contraction. The contraction should occur for approximately 5–10 seconds while the joint is fully extended.

Stretches and exercises to avoid

Some exercises and stretches have the potential to cause harm to an athlete, especially if done incorrectly. They may be safe for some but not all people because there is a moderate amount of anatomical variation between different people. A few of these anatomical differences can lead to serious consequences, so it is best for sports trainers to follow these general principles for stretching and warm-up exercises unless a specific recommendation has been made by an appropriate health professional following a proper assessment by them of an individual athlete:

- Extreme movements or stretching beyond any joint's normal range of motion can cause ligament strain and possible joint instability as well as muscle tears.

- For stretches involving the spine, special care should be taken. Athletes should try to maintain good posture so that the natural curves of the spine are maintained. They should also avoid extreme movements of the spine in any direction as these can potentially cause excessive strain or pressure on spinal structures such as joints and intervertebral discs.

- Full circular movements of the head or 'neck circling' movements should be avoided as the vertebrobasilar artery that supplies blood to part of the brain may be compromised when the neck is extended and rotated.

- Neck strengthening exercises that place body weight through the neck should be undertaken only with extreme caution and expert supervision. Although these exercises are used commonly in some martial arts, it is essential that this type of exercise is built up very gradually to allow muscles to develop adequately to provide protection to the neck.

- Generally, 'open kinetic chain' exercises, such as unsupported trunk bending into forward flexion or side bending, should be progressed slowly and only after supported 'closed kinetic chain' strengthening exercises, such as the front bridge, have been used to improve the power and control of muscles that provide stability to the area.

- Ballistic stretching is a term generally referring to high speed repetitive movements at the end of the range of movement, sometimes referred to as 'bouncing'. Ballistic stretching should be avoided as it carries a significant risk of muscle or tendon strain and does not produce any benefits that cannot be achieved with safer forms of stretching.

Cool-down and recovery

The cool-down is a gradual decrease in activity level designed to minimise excessive muscle tightening as the muscles cool and to maintain an adequate level of circulation for the purpose of reducing or 'flushing out' waste products such as lactic acid from the muscles. It can also be helpful in preventing a sudden drop in blood pressure after sport or exercise, which can lead to dizziness or fainting, by preventing the pooling of blood in the lower limbs that can occur if movement stops suddenly. The cool-down can involve light exercises such as jogging as well as gentle stretching exercises. In the cool-down phase, drinking water or suitable sports drinks and eating foods with carbohydrate and protein can also be helpful in reducing the effects of fatigue and possibly muscle tightness.

The cool-down session can also be a useful time for post-match debriefing as well as checking the players for injuries.

Full recovery after intense training or competition can take several days. Appropriate rest, a gradual return to exercise and nutrition and hydration strategies are all important parts of effective recovery programs. Incomplete recovery and overtraining have been shown to lead to increases in sports injury rates. The Sports Medicine Australia Clean Edge program has an online Over Training tool that athletes or their coaches can use to determine if they are over training (see www.cleanedge.com.au).

Prevention of re-injury

Once an injury has occurred there is a significantly increased risk of the athlete sustaining another injury. This is especially true if the initial injury is not managed properly, or if the athlete returns to training or competition before the injury has healed completely and full, correct rehabilitation has taken place. Therefore, to minimise the chance of re-injury, a properly structured return-to-sport program that gradually increases the load on the injured area is most important. This program needs to be conducted under the guidance of a health professional with expertise in sports injury rehabilitation. A comprehensive program will correct the underlying causes that contributed to the injury as well as correcting any damage caused by the injury. Sports trainers can assist with rehabilitation programs by ensuring the athlete complies fully with the prescribed rehabilitation program; this will include supervising the athlete's exercise program between visits to the treating health professional.

Introduction to sports massage

Sports trainers may benefit from undergoing additional training in basic sports massage. Athletes often use massage before events as part of their preparation and, sometimes, as part of the recovery process. To promote healing and recovery from exercise, many coaches and athletes seek massage based on the belief that it can increase muscle blood flow and aid in the clearance of swelling and removal of the waste products of muscle metabolism. It can also reduce tension and increase the athlete's sense of wellbeing. There is some evidence to support the use of massage in reducing post-exercise muscle soreness.

Massage before events is usually of a short duration and may be administered through clothing, depending on the time available and the athlete's preference. Massage might also occur while the athlete is sitting or standing, depending on the circumstances. Before events, it may be more or less vigorous, depending on whether relaxation or stimulation is the priority. Massage should not be used for injuries, especially in the acute stages, and it should only be prescribed by a health professional after a full assessment and diagnosis. Incorrect massage, particularly of muscles and joints, can cause or worsen injuries. Deep tissue massage should only be performed by people with comprehensive massage training.

When performing massage, sports trainers must ensure:

- they have the full consent of the athlete
- the athlete is appropriately draped to preserve modesty and maintain body temperature
- the person providing the massage is aware of their own body position to protect themselves from injury or strain associated with poor posture or overuse
- infection control practices and regulations are fully complied with.

Basic massage strokes

Comprehensive training in massage is valuable for a sports trainer, but some of the more basic massage strokes often used in sport include the following:

- Effleurage – a gliding technique applied to the superficial tissues. It is often used as the first and most basic form of massage and usually involves long, slow, gentle strokes. Effleurage can be performed with the open hand, fist or forearm. There are many variations of effleurage.

- Petrissage – techniques that involve the repetitive lifting, rolling, squeezing or compression of the soft tissues. A common petrissage technique is known as kneading and involves the alternate compression and lifting of the soft tissues.
- Tapotement – also known as tapping, it involves repeated percussive or tapping techniques. It is often used for stimulating effects.
- Friction – non-gliding movements of tissue over deeper tissues. They are usually performed with repetitive circular movements and are often used for deeper massage techniques.
- Vibration – techniques that utilise rhythmic tissue movements. They can be fast or slow, light or deep.

Protective equipment

Sports trainers should ensure that their athletes use suitable protective equipment during both training and competition. When examining protective equipment, the sports trainer should:

- ensure the equipment used complies with the rules of the sport
- ensure the equipment is specific and appropriate for the sport and for the size and age of the athlete
- check that it fits the athlete correctly
- regularly check and maintain protective equipment and ensure that worn or damaged equipment is replaced
- ensure the equipment used meets relevant quality and safety standards and that it is used according to the manufacturer's guidelines and the recommendations of the governing sporting body.

Preventive taping and bracing

Protective equipment can also include sports taping or braces designed to restrict or control certain joint or limb movements that could lead to musculo-skeletal injuries occurring during sport. This is covered more fully in Chapter 10.

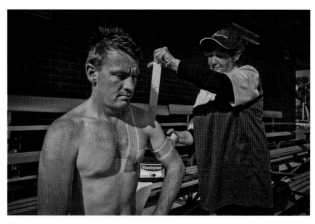

Figure 3.13 Taping for sports injury prevention

Shin and leg guards

Shin injuries are common in sports where there is a potential to be struck either by an opponent or by equipment such as a hockey stick or a hard ball. Properly fitted, well constructed leg or shin guards can prevent or minimise lower leg injuries. Different types of shin guards are used for different sports. For example, soccer shin pads tend to be light and flexible as opposed to hockey guards that have a firmer and more rigid construction. People in other sports, such as catchers in softball or baseball, have lower leg guards that cover the feet and knees, whereas a cricket batsman's leg guards extend above the knee.

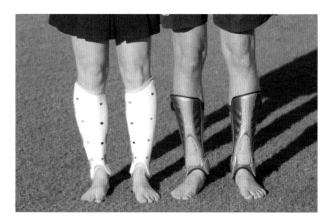

Figure 3.14 Shin pads for hockey (left) and soccer (right)

Wrist, elbow and knee guards

In sports such as rollerskating, rollerblading, snow skiing, snowboarding and skateboarding, athletes have a chance of falling onto hard surfaces so hard protective guards are often used to prevent injuries ranging from minor abrasions and other external wounds to more severe hard and soft tissue injuries. There are restrictions on the use of some types of hard protective guards in many sports.

Protective wrist guards are designed to protect the hand and wrist from injuries such as joint sprains or fractures resulting from a fall onto an outstretched hand.

Some types of knee protectors are designed to absorb impact forces from falls onto hard surfaces. They can be simply padded knee protectors, as used in sports such as volleyball, or they can also incorporate hard plastic components. Some knee protectors are also designed to protect the knee from excessive twisting movements. Professional advice as to type and fit is recommended for this type of knee protector.

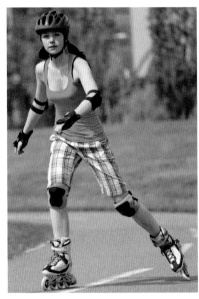

Figure 3.15 Wrist, elbow and knee guards

Shoulder padding and body protectors

In tackling and collision sports, shoulder protectors are sometimes used to protect the shoulder from impact injury. Sports where this is common include rugby union, rugby league and American football.

Padded body protectors help protect the trunk, particularly the chest area, from impact injury in sports such as fencing, softball and baseball. 'Boxes' or 'cups' for males in sports such as cricket are essential for protection of the external genitalia.

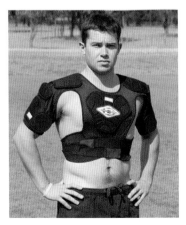

Figure 3.16 Shoulder protectors

Eye protection

Sports with a high risk of eye injury are those involving:

- a high speed ball or puck
- use of a bat, stick or racket
- close aggressive play with body contact or collision
- a combination of any of the above.

Some of these sports include squash, ice hockey, racquetball and lacrosse. Face and eye protection is recommended for all athletes in sports such as these.

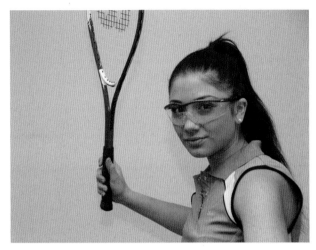

Figure 3.17 Sports eye protection

For athletes in competition who wear spectacles and participate in lower risk sports, normal street-wear spectacle frames with polycarbonate lenses give adequate and cosmetically acceptable protection for routine use. Clear polycarbonate frames and lenses are suggested for contact lens wearers and athletes who ordinarily do not wear glasses but participate in moderate to high-risk non-contact sports. They can be used in combination with a facemask or a helmet with face protection for additional protection in high-risk contact or collision sports.

If an athlete already has an eye problem or suffers from reduced vision, there is an increased risk of eye injury. Sports trainers and athletes should consult an optometrist for advice on vision requirements and protective eyewear specific to their sport. Some types of protective faceguards and eye protection can be worn over prescription eyewear.

Helmets/headgear

Helmets can reduce the risk of head injury in sports where the following are likely:

- high speed collisions (e.g. motor sports or cycling)
- potential for missile injuries (e.g. baseball or cricket)
- falls onto hard surfaces (e.g. ice hockey or skating).

Other protective headwear, such as headgear, may provide additional protection for the face and ears of athletes participating in sports such as the rugby codes.

It is important to note that helmets may not protect the athlete totally against many injuries, such as concussion and brain injury. Also, helmets may cause some athletes to become over confident and to take more risks in the mistaken belief that the helmet will protect them completely from injury.

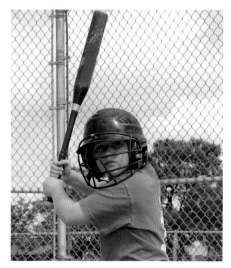

Figure 3.18 Sports helmet

Gloves

Protective gloves help prevent soft and hard tissue injuries of the fingers, hands and wrists. Padded gloves are used especially in sports with a hard, fast moving ball, such as baseball and cricket, or where there is a risk of falling to reduce abrasions, such as motor cycling. Gloves can also protect the hands from blisters and calluses, as well as cold weather-related circulatory problems. In sports such as golf, hockey and cricket, gloves are often used to improve grip and to reduce impact shock.

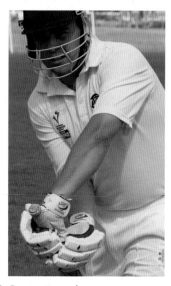

Figure 3.19 Protective gloves

Mouthguards

In any sport where there is a risk of a blow to the face or head from sporting equipment or from another player, athletes should wear a properly fitted mouthguard. Mouthguards act as a shock absorber for the teeth and jaw and, when properly fitted, reduce the risk of dental injuries.

Mouthguards should:
- fit the mouth accurately
- allow normal breathing and speech
- be custom designed and fitted by a qualified professional.

The most common types of mouthguards are:
1 Stock mouthguards – these are made of rigid plastic and are available at pharmacies and sports stores. They can be uncomfortable and interfere with normal breathing and speech. They are often not firmly secured and can offer a false sense of protection.

2 'Boil and bite' mouthguards – these are made from a thermoplastic material that is softened in hot water and then placed in the mouth to mould to the teeth as the guard is bitten. Like stock guards, they are cheap and their shape is easily deformed. They offer limited protection, they can be uncomfortable and they impair breathing and speech.

3 Custom-fitted mouthguards – these are made by a dental professional from shock-absorbing plastic cast from an impression of the teeth and gums of the individual athlete. The accurate fit and control of the thickness maximises the shock-absorbing effect of the mouthguard. They fit comfortably and do not interfere with breathing or speech. The National Health and Medical Research Council (NHMRC) recommends custom-made mouthguards for contact sports and the purchase and fitting of a new mouthguard at the beginning of each new competition season.

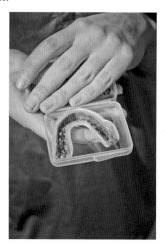

Figure 3.20 Custom-fitted mouthguard

Footwear

As well as having an effect on sporting performance, appropriate footwear is an important part of an athlete's protective equipment. Incorrect shoe types or poorly fitting or excessively worn shoes can lead to an increased chance of sports injury. Due to the number of footwear options available and the fact that different people have different foot types and movement patterns, athletes should ideally choose shoes based on the recommendation of a podiatrist or physiotherapist. Their recommendation will be based on an assessment of the athlete's foot type and lower limb biomechanics, as well as taking into account the specific demands of the sport and the type of playing surface.

Some of the main considerations for choosing athletic footwear are set out below.

TORSION OF THE SHOE

Some shoes can resist twisting movements more than others. The correct amount and location of shoe torsion required will vary between athletes depending on their foot type. For example, athletes whose feet excessively roll inwards when the foot contacts the ground (referred to as 'over pronation') generally will benefit from shoes that control or limit torsion while bearing weight. To test a shoe, grasp the heel and the front of the shoe near the ball of the foot and twist lengthways.

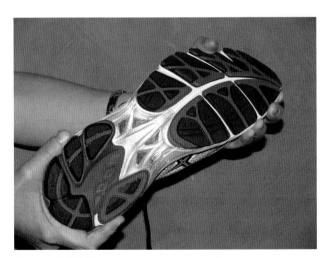

Figure 3.21 Testing torsion of the shoe

FLEXION OF THE SHOE

For most athletes, the forefoot flexibility of the shoe is important. To test a shoe, grasp the heel and toe of the shoe and push together. The shoe should bend at the ball of the foot.

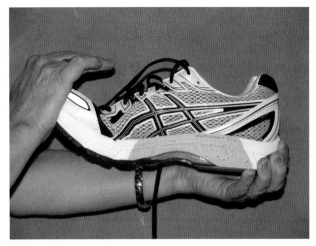

Figure 3.22 Testing forefoot flexibility of the shoe

MID-SOLE DENSITY

Mid-sole density can be tested as an indicator of the cushioning characteristics of the shoe. With your thumbs, compress the mid-sole. If it does not compress at all or is very stiff it may not absorb impact shock as well as a softer mid-sole. However, excessively soft cushioning might also be bad, depending on the athlete's foot type and the relevant sporting activity. If it compresses easily it may provide a high degree of cushioning initially, but this might also indicate a material that will compress more easily over time and not last well, especially in cheaper shoes. Some sports shoes have dual or multi-density mid-soles with different components that are designed to provide both cushioning and stability in a controlled way.

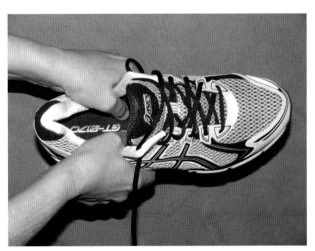

Figure 3.23 Testing shoe mid-sole density

HEEL COUNTER

The strength of the heel counter is related to the ability of the shoe to control the movement of the heel and the rear part of the foot. To test this, squash down on the heel counter with your thumb or squeeze it between your thumb and index finger. The material used in the heel counter can vary; cheap shoes often use materials such as cardboard that do not last well and are less effective in providing support.

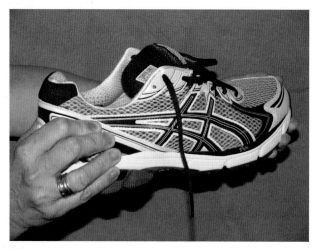

Figure 3.24 Testing heel counter of the shoe

TRACTION CHARACTERISTICS OF THE SOLE

The amount of grip between the sole of the shoe and the playing surface is an important consideration when choosing shoes for sport. Although insufficient grip can lead to increased slips and falls that lead to injury, too much traction or grip can also increase the likelihood of injury, especially twisting injuries of the lower limb. For this reason, the choice of sporting footwear needs to take into account local environmental conditions, the type of playing surfaces encountered and the demands of the sport. For example, a football boot with studs or cleats designed for soft lush surfaces may be uncomfortable and ineffective on hard grounds.

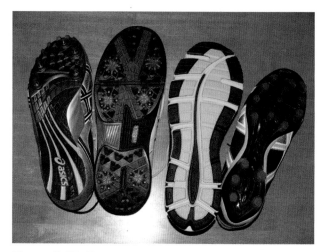

Figure 3.25 Footwear traction requirements vary among different sports and playing surfaces

Chapter Four

SPORTS NUTRITION

LEARNING OUTCOMES

Demonstrate a sound knowledge and understanding of basic nutrition for athletes.

1   Explain the general guidelines of food and nutrition for athletes.
2   Explain the relationship between nutrition and health to athletes.
3   Collect information on the different dietary strategies for optimising an athlete's body composition and sporting performance.
4   Explain the basic components of a balanced diet that fulfils the training needs of an athlete.
5   Explain the basic dietary requirements for an athlete's competition and recovery.
6   Interpret the nutritional information presented on food packaging.

ASSESSMENT OF OUTCOMES

Underpinning knowledge

Oral or written questions may be asked relating to nutrition and diet. You may also be asked to complete an online task or workbook with related activities.

Practical demonstration

You may be asked to explain the nutrition value of certain foods to your class or instructor.

Scenario

You may be asked to give an information session to athletes about dietary choices and their effect on sporting performance.

Introduction

Nutrition plays an important role in optimising an athlete's sporting performance. Good nutrition and hydration strategies are important before, during and after competition and training.

Effective, scientifically based nutrition and hydration strategies are an important part of maximising athletes' training benefits and performance during competition, so expert advice regarding nutrition and hydration from a sports dietitian is highly recommended. Unlike doctors and physiotherapists, dietitians rarely travel with sports teams so sports trainers have an especially important role in ensuring athletes comply with nutrition and hydration strategies that have been recommended to them by their dietitian or coach. Therefore, sports trainers should also develop a basic understanding of key sports nutrition principles and be able to recognise signs such as fatigue, cramps or reduced performance that indicate a referral to a dietitian might be appropriate.

Sometimes athletes who are interested in improving their performance develop nutritional habits that are ineffective and occasionally even dangerous. The sports person or athlete may be influenced by advertisements or articles in newspapers, magazines or health food stores that claim particular foods or supplements will improve athletic performance. Sports trainers are well placed to help athletes by encouraging them to seek expert advice from a sports health professional, such as a dietitian or doctor, before commencing non-standard eating plans or using dietary supplements.

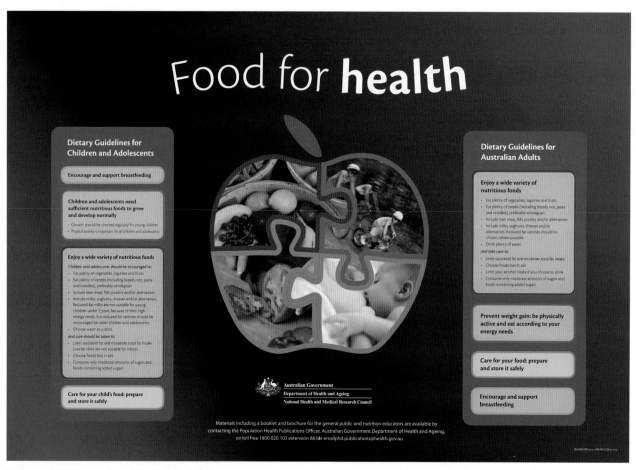

Figure 4.1 Australian Dietary Guidelines

Food for Health dietary guidelines

Dietary guidelines were released by the Australian Government Department of Health and Ageing and the National Health and Medical Research Council (NHMRC) in 2005 in their booklet, *Food for Health*. The guidelines promote healthy eating as well as the importance of leading a physically active lifestyle. The booklet is free to download from the NHMRC website (www.nhmrc.gov.au). It contains information and recommendations by experts about food groups and lifestyle patterns that promote good nutrition and health at each of the stages of a person's life when dietary needs are different.

The Dietary Guidelines for Australian Adults recommend that adults should:

- eat plenty of vegetables, legumes and fruits
- eat plenty of cereals (including breads, rice, pasta and noodles), preferably wholegrain
- include lean meat, fish, poultry and/or alternatives
- include milks, yoghurts, cheeses and/or alternatives. Reduced-fat varieties should be chosen, where possible
- drink plenty of water.

Adults should also take care to:

- limit saturated fat and moderate total fat intake
- choose foods low in salt
- limit their alcohol intake if they choose to drink
- consume only moderate amounts of sugars and foods containing added sugars.

The Dietary Guidelines for Children and Adolescents in Australia recommend that children and adolescents should enjoy a wide variety of nutritious foods and be encouraged to:

- eat plenty of vegetables, legumes and fruits
- eat plenty of cereals (including breads, rice, pasta and noodles), preferably wholegrain
- include lean meat, fish, poultry and/or alternatives
- include milks, yoghurts, cheese and/or alternatives. Reduced-fat milks are not suitable for young children under 2 years because of their high energy needs, but reduced-fat varieties should be encouraged for older children and adolescents
- choose water as a drink. Alcohol is not recommended for children.

In addition, care should be taken to:

- limit saturated fat and moderate total fat intake. Low-fat diets are not suitable for infants
- choose foods low in salt
- consume only moderate amounts of sugars and foods containing added sugars.

Energy sources and nutrients for sport

All foods and drinks contain nutrients. The major nutrients are carbohydrates, fat, protein, vitamins and minerals. In addition, dietary fibre and water are vital to life and help to regulate body processes. The sports trainer should appreciate how intricate and sophisticated our food is. Nutrients do not exist in isolation. For example, there is more to an orange than vitamin C and more to meat than protein. Food and fluids are a complex mixture of hundreds of nutrients. Therefore, it is wise to consume a wide variety of foods that provide a balance of all types of nutrients.

Carbohydrates, fat and protein are the energy-giving nutrients. During sport and physical activity, carbohydrates and fats provide the most energy. Protein is also a minor source of energy, especially in long duration activities when the stores of carbohydrate and fats are greatly depleted.

Carbohydrate

Carbohydrates are foods that are broken down by the body into simple sugars. Carbohydrate is the body's primary source of fuel during everyday activity and exercise. All cells in the human body require carbohydrate for energy. When carbohydrate is consumed it is broken down by the body and stored in muscles and the liver as glycogen. During physical activity, stored glycogen is broken down further to glucose, which provides the fuel for muscle contraction.

Glucose is the human body's, including the brain's, most economical energy source and preferred source of fuel. Because glycogen is broken down to glucose during exercise, glycogen stores need to be constantly replenished during and after exercise. High carbohydrate foods restore liver and muscle glycogen stores.

Low levels of carbohydrate may result in fatigue, ineffective training, reduced immunity and reduced muscle mass. The harder an athlete trains, the greater their daily carbohydrate needs.

Carbohydrate serves other important roles in the body, including preserving protein stores and facilitating fat metabolism and the proper functioning of the central nervous system.

Carbohydrate-rich foods include breads, cereals, rice, pasta and other grains, fruit, vegetables, legumes, milk and yoghurt. Sugar, lollies, soft drinks and honey also contain carbohydrate but contain few or no other nutrients.

Carbohydrates are grouped as either:

- simple carbohydrates – also known as simple sugars (e.g. white sugar)
- complex carbohydrates – also known as starches (e.g. bread and rice).

Carbohydrate-rich foods that are more slowly digested and absorbed are known as low glycaemic index (GI) foods. Low GI foods provide a slower and more sustained energy release. Examples of low GI foods are baked beans, pasta, oats and fruit. A combination of low and high GI foods may be appropriate depending on the type and duration of exercise or sport.

The actual amount of carbohydrate needed can vary significantly depending on the individual athlete's energy needs. To provide energy for a light to moderate training program, sports dietitians recommend that carbohydrate-rich foods should make up about half of the total energy intake. Athletes in heavy daily training may need to eat even higher levels. In order to meet these daily requirements every meal and snack should be based on carbohydrate-rich foods. A sports dietitian can work with an athlete to develop an eating plan that provides sufficient carbohydrate for their activity levels.

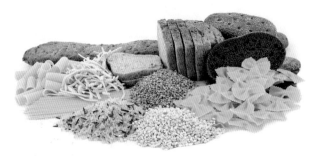

Figure 4.2 Nutritious carbohydrates

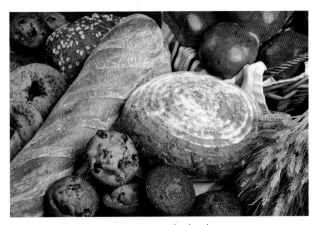

Figure 4.3 Less nutritious carbohydrates

Protein

Proteins are made up of amino acids, the building blocks of the human body. There are 20 types of amino acids, of which nine are essential for health, so a balanced diet is required to ensure all are available to the body. Proteins are crucial to the regulation and maintenance of our bodies. Proteins form important structures in the body, such as muscle tissue; they make up a key part of blood; and

they help regulate many body functions, such as blood clotting, fluid balance, hormone and enzyme production, visual processes and cell repair. If an athlete does not regularly eat sufficient protein, these and other metabolic processes may be affected. For example, the immune system may no longer function efficiently, which will increase the risk of infection. Protein may also provide a minor source of fuel for exercise.

Proteins fall into two classes:

1   Complete proteins (containing all nine essential amino acids) are found in animal-based protein products; for example, red meat, fish, poultry and dairy foods.

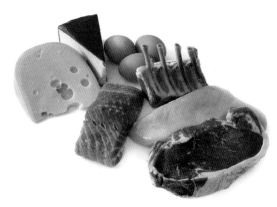

Figure 4.4 Complete proteins

2   Incomplete proteins (lacking in one or more essential amino acids) are found in plant-based protein products; for example, nuts, legumes, tofu, soy products, breads and cereals. However, protein foods can be 'complemented' to ensure all amino acids are obtained from the diet. This is especially important for vegetarian athletes.

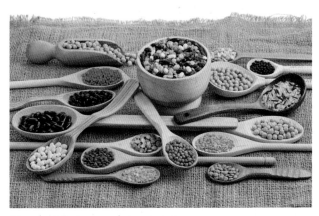

Figure 4.5 Incomplete proteins

Both strength and endurance athletes need additional protein due to increased muscle building and increased use of protein as a fuel, especially during endurance exercise. Most Australians eat 2–3 times as much protein as they need, and the typical high food intake of most athletes provides a more than adequate protein intake.

Some athletes, such as those in weight-restricted sports, fussy eaters or dieters, may be at risk of not eating enough protein. Poor protein intake may cause loss of muscle mass, slower recovery and serious health problems if continued for a long time.

Conversely, some athletes may be at risk of eating too much protein, particularly those wanting to increase muscle mass or those following certain types of high protein diets designed for weight loss. Some consequences of prolonged excessive protein intake include increased progression of preexisting kidney disease, atherogenic effects, increased urinary calcium excretion and increased fluid loss.

Fats (lipids)

Fats also play a vital role in the body and the food we eat. Fats provide a source of energy and reserve, protect vital organs, provide thermal insulation and are a carrier of fat-soluble vitamins (A, D, E and K). Fats (lipids) contain more than twice the energy per gram as proteins and carbohydrates. There are several types of compounds that can be classified as fats but triglycerides form the major component of food-based fat that is consumed and stored in the body by humans.

Fats are generally classified into two main groups:

1 Saturated fats (solid at room temperature) – sources include animal-based foods (e.g. fat found in meat and poultry, dairy foods, butter, cream, many fast foods and snack products). These fats should be limited in the diet. An individual concerned about heart health should choose lean meats and reduced-fat dairy products and limit intake of 'treat type' foods.

2 Unsaturated fats (liquid at room temperature), monounsaturated and polyunsaturated – sources include plant-based foods and fish foods (e.g. canola, olive and sunflower oils, margarine and the fats contained in avocado, nuts and seeds, salmon and tuna). Unsaturated fats should make up the majority of an individual's fat intake.

Excess body fat stores may impair performance. Often athletes eat too much fat at the expense of carbohydrate and, therefore, may not adequately replenish glycogen stores. For athletes and the general population fat should contribute less than 30% of energy consumed. By making healthy, low-fat, high-carbohydrate and protein food choices at all meals and snacks, performance can be maximised.

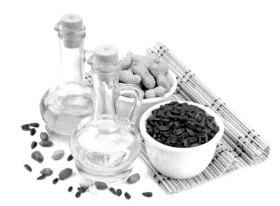

Figure 4.6 Unsaturated fats

Vitamins

Although vitamins provide no energy, they aid in many energy-releasing reactions in the body. In this way, vitamins promote growth, development and maintenance of body tissues. For a substance to be classified as a vitamin, its absence from the diet for a defined period of time must produce deficiency signs and symptoms that, if caught in time, could be cured when the substance is reintroduced to the diet.

There are two types of vitamins:

1 fat soluble (absorbed and transported by fats) – vitamins A, D, E and K

2 water soluble (absorbed and transported by water) – B group vitamins and vitamin C.

Vitamin A

Vitamin A is needed for healthy growth and healthy skin and eyes. It is found in oily fish, vegetables (especially carrots and spinach), liver and dairy products.

B group vitamins

The B group vitamins include:

- thiamine
- riboflavin
- niacin
- folate
- pantothenic acid
- biotin
- B-6
- B-12.

B group vitamins, which are found mainly in cereals, leafy vegetables, liver, eggs and milk, are needed to help release energy from our food, for healthy growth and healthy skin.

Vitamin C

Vitamin C is found in fresh fruit and vegetables. It helps maintain proper cell structure and function. It cannot be stored in the body for extended periods and needs to be ingested regularly.

Vitamin D

Vitamin D is found mostly in oily fish, eggs and dairy products. It is made in small amounts by the effects of the sun on the skin. It controls the amounts of minerals available for bone formation.

Vitamin E

Vitamin E is found in many foods containing plant oils and wholegrain cereals. It is needed for cell growth and wound healing.

Vitamin K

Vitamin K is found in leafy green vegetables and liver. It contributes to blood clotting, which stops blood loss from a wound.

Minerals

Minerals contribute to body compounds, water balance and body growth and development. At all levels of body function (cellular, tissue, organ and whole body), minerals play an important role.

They are classified generally into two categories:
1 major minerals (100 mg or more required per day) – for example, sodium, potassium and calcium
2 trace minerals (less than 100 mg required per day) – for example, iron and zinc.

Sodium

Sodium is readily absorbed by the human body and plays a key role in retaining water, assisting nerve function and allowing absorption of other nutrients. Low levels of sodium in the body can result in muscle cramping, nausea, vomiting and dizziness. Extremely low levels can lead to shock and coma. This is particularly relevant to athletes as a low-sodium diet coupled with excessive perspiration can seriously deplete the body of sodium. High levels of sodium in the body are associated with high blood pressure and hypertension. Approximately one-half of the sodium a person consumes is added during cooking or at the table. The remainder is often added to food during manufacture and processing.

Potassium

Potassium performs many of the same functions as sodium, such as maintaining fluid balance and assisting nerve function. Low levels of potassium in the body can affect heart function. Fruits, vegetables, milk, whole grains, dried beans and meats are all good sources of potassium.

Calcium

Calcium plays a major role in the body in the formation and maintenance of bone tissue. It also helps with several other functions such as blood clotting, transmission of nerve impulses, muscle contraction and cell metabolism. Dairy products provide the richest sources of calcium.

Iron

Iron is found in red blood cells, muscle cells and in cell mitochondria. It is therefore important for oxygen transportation and synthesis in the body. Meat, poultry, seafood, dry beans, eggs, nuts and whole grains are all good sources of iron. Athletes need to pay particular attention to ensure they maintain adequate levels of iron in their diet. Iron deficiency is associated with tiredness, headaches, irritability and depression.

Zinc

An adequate level of zinc is necessary to support many body functions. These include:
- DNA synthesis
- protein metabolism, wound healing and growth
- sexual organ development
- bone development
- insulin function and storage
- cell membrane structure and function.

Generally, protein-rich foods are high in zinc. Red meat and shellfish are the best sources of zinc, but it can be found in other foods such as wheat germ, wholegrain cereals, eggs and nuts.

Water

Water is second only to oxygen in importance to the human body. Without water, all biological processes necessary for life would cease in a few days. Many nutrients, including minerals, exist in the body dissolved in water. Water serves several functions in the body; it controls body temperature, lubricates joints, protects organs, removes wastes and carries blood cells and nutrients around the body.

Each day, the human body needs to replace about two litres of fluid to balance normal daily losses. Additional fluid is required to cover sweat losses during exercise and physical activity. An individual's requirement increases in hot and humid environments and with increased salt, protein, fibre, alcohol and caffeine intake.

If an individual does not adequately replace their fluid losses, dehydration will result. The signs and symptoms of dehydration include:

- increased perception of effort
- increased body temperature and heart rate
- reduced mental function
- poor concentration and coordination
- fatigue or dizziness
- nausea
- vomiting
- headache
- muscle or stomach cramps
- thirst
- dry mouth
- dark yellow urine.

There are many options available to athletes to replenish fluid and electrolytes lost from the body. Water alone is an effective drink for fluid replacement in low-intensity and short-duration sports. However, during high-intensity and endurance sports, carbohydrate and electrolyte intake generally improves or sustains performance.

Electrolytes, such as sodium and potassium (see page 42), are lost in sweat and need to be replaced *during* extended or *after* prolonged exercise. Sodium stimulates thirst receptors causing the athlete to drink more and encourages greater fluid retention.

Sports drinks

Sports drinks are specially formulated drinks designed to improve performance during exercise and/or recovery after exercise. Sports drinks contain carbohydrate and electrolytes designed to maintain and replenish stores consumed during exercise. Depending on the individual's needs and the type of sport or exercise, sports drinks may be useful before, during and after exercise.

An ideal sports drink for consumption before sport and exercise is typically made up of 4–8% carbohydrate, contains electrolytes such as sodium and tastes good to encourage consumption. Some may also contain caffeine, which can improve performance, although excessive levels of caffeine can also potentially have a dehydrating effect that can negatively affect performance. Sports drinks for recovery usually contain protein as well as carbohydrate.

Athletes consuming large quantities of sports drinks for prolonged periods should pay extra attention to dental hygiene as sports drinks are highly acidic and may lead to tooth decay. Rinsing the mouth with water immediately after consuming a sports drink may reduce these effects. For more information on hydration, see Chapter 7.

Dietary fibre

Dietary fibre is a plant-based substance that is undigested by the body. It plays an important role in an individual's diet. Dietary fibre aids in the removal of unwanted chemicals from the intestine, prevents constipation, aids in weight control, helps prevent intestinal cancers and aids in the control of blood sugar and cholesterol levels.

Dietary fibre can be classified as either:

- insoluble fibre (does not dissolve in water) – for example, whole grains, bran and corn
- soluble fibre (dissolves or swells in water) – for example, fruit and vegetables, oats, barley and legumes.

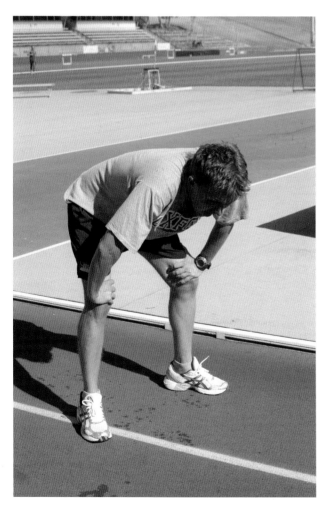

Figure 4.7 The effects of dehydration

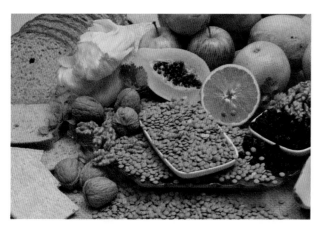

Figure 4.8 Dietary fibre

It is beneficial to include both types of fibre in the diet. Insoluble fibre assists in removing waste from the intestine and reduces the risk of constipation and bowel cancer. Soluble fibre softens bowel motions and assists in reducing high blood cholesterol levels.

Pre-event and recovery nutrition

Pre-event nutrition

An athlete needs to have adequate carbohydrate fuel stores in the muscles and liver. If athletes are training or competing each day, particularly for more than one session each day, it is crucial that they constantly restore their muscle glycogen levels. The carbohydrate foods eaten in the hours immediately before sport can help replenish these glycogen levels.

An athlete's normal overnight fast will lower liver glycogen stores, which in turn can reduce their endurance. Eating a carbohydrate-rich meal or snack before sport gives them a much better chance of maintaining normal blood glucose levels and enhancing both physical and mental performance.

Dehydration in sport can reduce an athlete's performance. In most situations, sweat loss during exercise is much greater than the amount of fluid an athlete can replace during a session. Athletes need to start the session well hydrated to minimise the impending fluid deficit; this will mean drinking a substantial amount of fluid with the pre-event meal or snack and having another drink 10–15 minutes before the start of their workout.

Athletes who easily get stomach upsets or have sensitive intestines and find it difficult to eat solid food before competition should try choosing low-fibre carbohydrate foods or liquid meals. A reduced fibre intake can help prevent bloating, diarrhoea and stomach discomfort. Liquid meals such as commercial high-carbohydrate drink supplements and homemade fruit smoothies made from milk and fruit allow an athlete to fuel up without creating a feeling of being uncomfortably full.

It is recommended that the pre-event meal be consumed 2–4 hours before competition. This may vary according to the type and timing of the event. The athlete will need enough time for the meal to be emptied from the stomach. Low-fat, high-carbohydrate meals and snacks empty the quickest from the stomach. Anxiety can slow stomach emptying. If an athlete is nervous before sport, they should allow more time for their stomach to empty. It is important that the timing is right for gastric comfort – they should be neither too full at the start of the event nor hungry late in the session. For events in the morning, an athlete might schedule their breakfast 2–3 hours prior to the event. In the case of a very early start, most athletes prefer to have a lighter snack 1–2 hours before the event and a larger supper the night before. Those competing later in the day may choose to eat their normal meals in the earlier part of the day and then have a light snack 1–2 hours prior to the event.

Nutrition during and after exercise

If the sport or training lasts no longer than an hour, an athlete should perform well without having to replace fuels until they have finished. Their next meals, if well chosen, will replace all the fuel they have used. However, as the athlete will start sweating and losing fluid very soon after they start exercise, fluid must be replaced as soon as possible during sport, otherwise even minor dehydration will decrease their performance.

If the sport or training takes longer than an hour, an athlete may benefit from consuming some carbohydrates during sport in addition to fluids; for example, sports drinks. The decision will depend on:

- the intensity of the exercise (higher intensity burns glycogen faster)
- the duration (the longer the event, the more glycogen burned)
- the ambient temperature (the hotter it is, the more quickly glycogen will be burned)
- what they have eaten before sport (more pre-event carbohydrate means more available glycogen).

Carbohydrate consumed during an event may improve endurance by:

- sparing muscle glycogen – in low-intensity exercise the carbohydrates taken during the event can be remade into glycogen for later use
- maintaining blood glucose (sugar) at normal levels during moderate to high-intensity exercise and providing extra fuel for muscles, thereby delaying fatigue.

Water is good for replacing fluid losses after sport. However, sports drinks have a number of advantages, including a taste that encourages better fluid intake and the addition of carbohydrates for glycogen fuel replacement. Glycogen replacement is beneficial if the event lasts an hour or more. Some sports drinks also have protein to assist in recovery.

To take advantage of the body's desire to replace glycogen stores after exercise, dietitians recommend that a post-event snack be eaten within 2 hours after exercise, although the first 30 minutes may be the most crucial. The body replaces glycogen at the quickest rate when carbohydrate foods and drinks are eaten soon after exercise. This becomes very important when an athlete trains or competes two or more times a day and they need to replace glycogen quickly. A larger meal can be consumed later, when an athlete has cooled down and feels more comfortable. Muscle glycogen can generally be replaced at 5% per hour, so it takes about 20 hours to replace an empty glycogen fuel tank.

As a guide, a recovery meal or snack should:
- be high in carbohydrate
- be moderate in protein
- include plenty of fluids.

For most events, the emphasis is on replacing carbohydrates and fluids. Athletes who find it difficult to eat solid food after exercise should try liquid sources of nutrition. Liquid meals, such as commercial high-carbohydrate drink supplements and homemade fruit smoothies, fruit juice and sports drinks, help an athlete to refuel and replace fluids even when they are not hungry.

It is recommended that an athlete eat 1–2 g of carbohydrate per kilogram of body weight in the 2 hours after exercise. This will equate to between 50 and 160 g of carbohydrate for most athletes.

There may be some good reasons for choosing carbohydrate foods that are also good sources of other nutrients, such as protein and vitamins or minerals. Speedy intake of these nutrients may assist in a variety of recovery activities, such as rebuilding protein or assisting the immune function.

Hydration

Encourage drinking before, during and after exercise. As well as decreasing sporting performance,

dehydration contributes to fatigue and can increase an athlete's likelihood of developing cramps, heat stress and heat stroke.

Athletes should not use thirst as an indicator of dehydration. Once an athlete feels thirsty, this is an indicator that they are already too dehydrated to perform at their best. Clear urine is a good indicator of an adequate level of hydration.

Exercise in hot or humid weather results in additional sweating, which increases fluid loss and increases the likelihood of dehydration.

To avoid dehydration athletes should start drinking plenty of fluids several hours before starting exercise. A good guide is to drink at least 500 mL 1 hour before exercise and at least 150 mL every 15 minutes during exercise. Once exercise or sport is finished athletes should drink liberally to rehydrate adequately.

The SMA Smartplay 'Drink Up' brochure provides a good summary of useful information about hydration (www.smartplay.com.au).

Food labelling

Food labels contain useful information to help an athlete make choices about food. The nutrition information panel indicates the quantities of various nutrients a food contains per serve, as well as per 100 g or 100 mL. It is best to use the 'per 100 g' or 'per 100 mL' to compare similar products, because the size of one 'serving' may differ between manufacturers.

Under labelling laws introduced in Australia in 2003, virtually all manufactured foods must show a nutrition information panel, which allows individuals to compare similar products and choose the one that suits their needs. There are a few exceptions: for example, foods in very small packages, foods such as herbs and spices, tea and coffee, foods sold unpackaged (if a claim is not made on the label) and foods made and packaged at the point of sale. Nutrition information panels provide information on the levels of energy (kilojoules), protein, total fat, saturated fat, carbohydrate, sugars and sodium, as well as any other nutrients, such as fibre, potassium, calcium and iron, about which a claim is made on the label.

NUTRITION INFORMATION

Serving Size: 30g (2 biscuits) Servings per pack: 42	AVG PER SERVE	TOTAL DAILY INTAKE (DI#)	AVG PER 100g
ENERGY	447kJ	8700kJ	1490kJ
	107Cal	2080Cal	356Cal
PROTEIN	3.7g	50g	12.4g
FAT – TOTAL	0.4g	70g	1.4g
– SATURATED FAT	0.1g	24g	0.3g
CARBOHYDRATE – TOTAL	20.1g	310g	67g
– SUGARS	1.0g	90g	3.3g
DIETARY FIBRE	3.3g	30g	11.0g
SODIUM	87mg	2300mg	290mg

	PER SERVE	%RDI* PER SERVE	PER 100g
POTASSIUM	102mg		340mg
ZINC	1.8mg	15%RDI*	6.0mg
IRON	3.0mg	25%RDI*	10.0mg
MAGNESIUM	32mg	10%RDI*	107mg
THIAMIN (Vitamin B1)	0.55mg	50%RDI*	1.83mg
RIBOFLAVIN (Vitamin B2)	0.43mg	25%RDI*	1.4mg
NIACIN (Vitamin B3)	2.5mg	25%RDI*	8.3mg
FOLATE	100µg	50%RDI**	333µg

What is Total DI & RDI?

#DI – Total Daily Intakes are based on an average adult diet of 8700kJ. Your daily intakes may be higher or lower depending on your energy needs.
*RDI – Recommended Dietary Intake.
** = 1 serve provides 25% of the folate RDI for women of childbearing age.

Ingredients: Wholegrain **wheat** (97%), raw sugar, salt, **barley** malt extract, minerals (zinc gluconate, iron), vitamins (niacin, thiamin, riboflavin, folate).
Contains cereals containing gluten.

Figure 4.9 Australian and New Zealand food labelling

Food products will also have a list of ingredients on the package. All ingredients must be listed in decreasing order by weight. Therefore:

- the ingredient listed first is present in the largest amount
- the ingredient listed last is present in the smallest amount.

Where there are very small amounts of multicomponent ingredients (less than 5%), it is permitted to list 'composite' ingredients only; for example, it may say 'chocolate' (rather than cocoa, cocoa butter and sugar) in a chocolate chip cookie or say 'tomato sauce' (rather than tomatoes, capsicum, onions and herbs) on a frozen pizza. This does not apply to any additive or allergen, which must be listed however small the amount.

Foods with a shelf life of less than 2 years must have a 'best before' date. It may still be safe to eat those foods after that date but they may have lost quality and some nutritional value. Those foods that should not be consumed after a certain date for health and safety reasons must have a 'use by' date. An exception is bread, which can be labelled with a 'baked on' or 'baked for' date if its shelf life is less than 7 days.

Food additives serve many different purposes, including making processed food easier to use or ensuring food is preserved safely. They may come from a synthetic or a natural source. For example, emulsifiers prevent salad dressings from separating into layers and preservatives help to keep food safe or fresh longer. All food additives must have a specific use, must have been assessed and approved by Food Standards Australia and New Zealand for safety and must be used in the lowest possible quantity that will achieve their purpose. Food additives must be identified, usually by a number, and included in the ingredients list. This allows people who may be sensitive to food additives to avoid them.

Note: Some of the information on sports nutrition was obtained from fact sheets available on the Sports Dietitians Australia website (http://www.sportsdietitians.com.au). Please refer to this website for further information.

Chapter Five

DRUGS IN SPORT

LEARNING OUTCOMES

Demonstrate a sound knowledge and understanding of permitted and prohibited drug regimens in sport.

1   Demonstrate non-judgemental approaches to drug use.
2   Demonstrate working within the defined roles and responsibilities as a sports trainer with regard to drugs.
3   Demonstrate a harm-minimisation approach to work and a range of activities that support this.
4   Describe athletes' needs and rights including duty of care.

ASSESSMENT OF OUTCOMES

Underpinning knowledge

Oral or written questions may be asked relating to drugs and prohibited substances and methods in sport. You may also be asked to complete an online task or workbook with related activities.

Practical demonstration

You may be asked to explain the effects certain drugs have on athletes and describe prohibited methods of doping to your class or instructor.

Scenario

You may be asked to give an information session to athletes about drug use in your particular sport.

Introduction

The reasons for drug or substance use and abuse are many and varied. Drugs and other prohibited methods may be used recreationally, to enhance performance, to inflict intentional self-harm or to attempt suicide. All drugs, whether legal or illegal, have some side effects and the legal status in no way reflects the amount of harm they may cause. Side effects depend on the type of drug, the amount taken, the metabolism of the person using the drug and whether the drug is used in conjunction with any other drugs.

Drug use in sport is more than anabolic steroids or the deliberate use of drugs and substances to improve performance. It also involves medications used to treat illness and injury and the use of social drugs such as alcohol and tobacco. When people talk about drug use in sport they tend to be referring to elite athletes who use various drugs to improve their performance by building muscles and strength. However, the use of drugs by sportsmen and sportswomen can encompass broader issues such as the ethics of drug use in sport and the role of regulatory bodies. It is not a new concept in sport. History shows that taking substances to improve performance has been going on since long before the beginning of the modern Olympics but, in the past century, the use of stimulants and other anabolic agents such as steroids to improve athletic performance has become more widespread.

What is a drug?

A drug is any substance that, when it enters the body, changes the way a person's mind and/or body functions.

General classification of drugs

Drugs can be classified by either the effect they have on the body or their availability to the population (legal status).

Effects

STIMULANTS

These are drugs that have the ability to increase activity in the central nervous system. They often make a person feel more alert and confident but may also cause overstimulation.

Stimulant drugs can have the following effects on the human body:

- increase alertness and mask the signs of fatigue
- produce feelings of euphoria and enhanced wellbeing
- cause anxiety and bizarre behaviour
- increase heart rate
- increase blood pressure
- increase respiratory rate
- constrict blood vessels
- dilate pupils
- suppress appetite
- cause insomnia.

Some common stimulant drugs include:

- caffeine – found in coffee, tea, cola soft drinks, caffeine-containing 'energy' drinks and fatigue-reduction medications
- nicotine – found in tobacco products
- amphetamines – for example, speed, ecstasy, benzedrine, dexedrine
- cocaine – made from the erythroxylon coca bush (also known as coke)
- crack – a crystallised freebase form of cocaine.

DEPRESSANTS

These are drugs that have the ability to slow down activity in the central nervous system. They have a calming and relaxing effect on the body in low doses and adversely affect coordination and concentration. In large doses, depressants can cause generalised incoordination, slurred speech, nausea and vomiting and may cause unconsciousness from reduced breathing and heart rates. Different classes of depressant should not be taken together as their effects are exacerbated, increasing the risk of overdose.

Depressant drugs can have the following effects on the human body:

- analgesic effects (pain reduction)
- anaesthetic effects (loss of sensation)
- decreased heart rate
- decreased respiratory rate
- relief from anxiety
- sedation
- feelings of euphoria and increased wellbeing.

Some common depressant drugs include:
- alcohol
- narcotic analgesics – found in opium products; for example, heroin, morphine and codeine
- general anaesthetics – surgical anaesthetics and inhaled anaesthetics; for example, nitrous oxide and methoxyflurane
- sedative hypnotics – for example, barbiturates, benzodiazepines (tranquillisers)
- cannabis – found in the *Cannabis sativa* plant (also called hashish or marijuana).

HALLUCINOGENS

Hallucinogenic (or psychedelic) drugs alter a person's perception of reality. They affect all the senses and can also markedly alter mood and thought. Hallucinogenic drugs can have a variety of effects on the body and are subjective to the drug user. Reactions can range from feelings of dread and terror (a bad trip) to extreme euphoria.

Some common hallucinogenic drugs include:
- marijuana/hashish (in high doses), found in the *Cannabis sativa* plant; it also has depressant effects in small amounts
- LSD (lysergic acid diethylamide), made in home laboratories
- mescaline, found in products made from the Mexican peyote cactus
- psilocybin, found in products made from the psilocybe and conocybe mushrooms; commonly known as magic mushrooms
- PCP (phencyclidine), chemically produced in a laboratory; commonly known as angel dust
- MDMA (methylenedioxymethamphetamine), a stimulant chemically produced in a laboratory; commonly known as ecstasy.

Availability of drugs

ILLEGAL DRUGS

Some drugs are banned for use by the general public as they can have dangerous consequences if not used for their intended purpose, whereas others are classified as illegal or illicit because they are deemed to have little or no medicinal value. Illicit drugs have no quality controls dictating their manufacture, price or distribution. As a consequence, the strength, purity and availability of a particular drug are unpredictable and can result in considerable harm to the user. Unintentional overdose may result from the unpredictable purity of drugs, such as the purity of heroin, and additives to any illicit drugs can be poisonous, which may result in injury and even death.

LEGAL DRUGS

The majority of the population can purchase these drugs. Certain laws may restrict their sale to people of a certain age (e.g. alcohol and tobacco). They can also be available 'over the counter' or via a medical practitioner's prescription.

PRESCRIPTION DRUGS

These drugs can only be purchased with a doctor's prescription and they are used to treat specific health problems or conditions. They should only be used for their intended purpose (e.g. antibiotics for infection, tranquillisers for anxiety or panic disorders and psychosis) and at the dosage indicated.

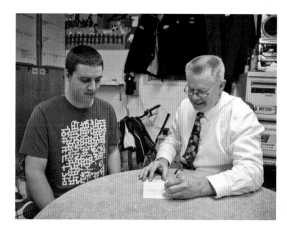

Figure 5.1 Prescription issued by a doctor

OVER-THE-COUNTER DRUGS

These drugs can be purchased from shops or pharmacies without a prescription. They are used to promote health (e.g. vitamin and mineral supplements, herbal and homeopathic products etc) or to treat minor pain and illness. They can still cause harmful effects if not used for their intended purpose (e.g. mild analgesics such as aspirin and paracetamol can be dangerous in high doses).

All drugs and medications, including prescription drugs and those available over the counter, can have serious side effects. These side effects may become a problem when the body is placed under the additional stress of physical activity.

Why athletes take drugs

Over the course of history, some athletes have tried to gain an advantage over their competitors with the use of drugs and other performance-enhancing substances.

Why do athletes take drugs? Unfortunately, there has been limited research into answering this question, but there are a number of possible reasons:
- a belief that their competitors are taking drugs
- a determination to do anything possible to achieve success

- direct or indirect pressure from coaches, parents and peers
- pressure from governing or sporting authorities
- lack of access to legal and natural methods to enhance performance (e.g. nutrition and psychological support)
- community attitudes and expectations regarding success and performance
- financial rewards
- influence from the media in facilitating these expectations and rewards.

The reasons for drug taking vary among athletes, but a combination of the above factors is present in most athletes who take drugs.

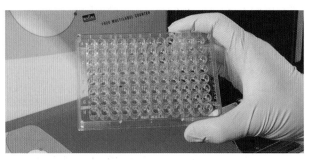

Figure 5.2 Drug testing at the Australian Drug Testing Laboratory

Which athletes can be tested for drugs?

Any person who represents their sport at a national or international level is eligible to be drug tested. Some sporting organisations (e.g. state/territory sporting institutes, Australian Institute of Sport and state/territory organisations) may have specific anti-doping policies and may also subject their athletes to testing at a state/territory level. Athletes should first seek information regarding their sport's anti-doping policy from the specific national or state/territory sporting organisation or institute. Testing occurs in and out of competition for substances and doping methods prohibited by a particular sport. Athletes and the people who support them should be educated on issues relating to drugs in sport, including:

- which drugs are permitted
- drug testing procedures
- athletes' rights and responsibilities.

Doping

Doping is the deliberate or inadvertent (accidental) use by athletes of banned substances or methods that may enhance performance.

Inadvertent doping

Inadvertent doping occurs when an athlete uses a medication to treat an illness without realising that it contains a banned substance and, consequently, returns a positive drug test result. In this situation, even though the athlete is not taking the drug deliberately to enhance performance, a positive test may still result in sanctions. A policy of strict liability exists in elite sports whereby athletes are responsible for any prohibited substance detected in their sample.

Some examples of medications that contain banned drugs are some cough suppressants and cold and flu medications. In most cases, there is another medication that does not contain a banned drug that can be used to treat the illness.

Prohibited substances and procedures

The substances and methods that are banned by most national sporting organisations are based on those banned by the World Anti Doping Agency (WADA). The majority of sporting organisations subscribe to the codes outlined by WADA, especially for one-off events such as national and international championships.

Most sports adopt the WADA codes to determine prohibited substances and methods for those athletes eligible to be drug tested. It is important that sports trainers and athletes regularly check with their national sporting organisation to confirm any variances to the WADA Anti Doping Code.

Prohibited classes of substances

The following classes of substances are prohibited:

- **Stimulants** – not all stimulants are prohibited and some are only prohibited in high doses. Contact your sporting organisation for specific information on prohibited stimulants.
- **Narcotic analgesics** – not all narcotic analgesics are prohibited and some are only prohibited in high doses. Contact your sporting organisation for specific information on prohibited narcotic analgesics.
- **Anabolic agents**.
- **Anabolic androgenic steroids (AAS)** are synthetic compounds based on the structure of testosterone. They are banned in sport because anabolic agents are prescribed for medical use only. Use of anabolic agents may enhance an athlete's performance, giving them an unfair advantage. Another concern is the serious medical side effects for the user. The amount of tissue building and masculinising that occurs as a result of taking one of these

drugs may be dependent on many different factors, including gender, diet, genetic characteristics, exercise and age.

- **Beta-2 agonists** work to open the airways in the lungs. For athletes with mild asthma, inhaled beta-2 agonists are typically used and readily available over the counter in all Australian states and territories. Asthma treatment is a particularly sensitive issue in sport. The list of acceptable treatments is subject to change. It is advisable to check with your sporting organisation or the Australian Sports Anti-Doping Authority (ASADA) to confirm suitable treatment.

- **Diuretics** are a family of drugs that promote urination. They are used to reduce water accumulation associated with heart failure, cirrhosis and corticosteroid therapy, as well as to treat high blood pressure. They are included on the banned drugs list because they can be misused to lose weight quickly for sports that have weight categories, or to increase the rate of urine production and elimination. Diluting urine makes it more difficult to detect the presence of a prohibited performance-enhancing drug. The side effects include dehydration, which can lead to fatal kidney and heart failure.

- **Peptide hormones, mimetics and analogues** – peptide hormones are substances that are produced by glands in the body and, after circulating through the blood, they can affect other organs and tissues to change bodily functions. They serve as messengers between different organs that stimulate various bodily functions such as growth, behaviour and sensitivity to pain. They are included on the banned substances list because they stimulate the production of naturally occurring hormones, increase muscle growth and strength and increase the production of red blood cells to improve the ability of the blood to carry oxygen. Mimetics and analogues are substances that act as masking agents, making the detection of banned substances more difficult.

Prohibited procedures

The following procedures are prohibited:

- Blood doping – this refers to various techniques used to increase the oxygen-carrying capacity of blood. Recently, recombinant human erythropoietin, more commonly known as EPO, has been the drug of choice.

- Administering artificial oxygen carriers or plasma expanders.

- Pharmacological, chemical and physical manipulation – athletes sometimes try to cover up the use of banned substances. Some of the methods used are drawing off urine from the bladder with a tube (catheterisation), using chemicals to hide performance-enhancing drugs (masking agents) and the swapping of urine samples.

Classes of prohibited substances in certain circumstances

Some substances may be allowable for use in some sports but prohibited in others.

Some of the substances that are prohibited in certain circumstances are set out below. For example, use of beta blocker drugs during competition is banned by many sports, though shooting and archery also ban their use outside of competition as well. Furthermore, whether these substances may be used by sports people will also depend in some cases on variations in local laws, so the athlete must both consult with their doctor as to their health effects and be aware of the legislation in place in the country or state they are competing in.

- Alcohol is a depressant drug that enters the bloodstream and dissolves in the water of the blood. The blood carries the alcohol throughout the body. The alcohol from the blood then enters and dissolves in the water inside each tissue of the body (except fat tissue, as alcohol cannot dissolve in fat). Once inside the tissues, alcohol exerts its depressant effects on the body.

- Cannabinoids are a group of chemicals that activate the body's cannabinoid receptors and act as either depressants or hallucinogens on the body. Currently, there are three general types of cannabinoids:
  - Herbal cannabinoids occur uniquely in the cannabis plant.
  - Endogenous cannabinoids are produced in the bodies of humans and other animals.
  - Synthetic cannabinoids are similar compounds produced in the laboratory.

- Local anaesthetics are drugs that cause a complete loss of feeling in a part of the body but do not cause a loss of consciousness (as occurs in general anaesthesia). Local anaesthetics work by blocking the nerves from a part of the body so that pain signals cannot reach the brain.

- Glucocorticosteriods (e.g. cortisone) are powerful anti-inflammatory agents. They may be administered in a variety of ways to treat chronic inflammatory conditions such as arthritis, asthma, inflamed joints and allergic reactions.

■ Beta-blockers 'block' the effects of adrenaline on the body's beta-receptors, which are nerve receptors found in many organs including the heart, lungs and blood vessels. Beta-blockers thereby reduce the heart rate and blood pressure as well as having effects on several other body systems.

The therapeutic use of banned medications (Therapeutic Use Exemptions)

In some cases, an athlete must use a medication that does contain a banned drug for a genuine therapeutic reason, such as the medical treatment of an illness. In these cases, it is suggested that athletes who are subject to doping control should take the following steps:

1 Check with their doctor to ensure there is no suitable alternative medication that could be taken that does not contain a substance on the Prohibited List.

2 Contact their national sporting organisation to identify whether they may be eligible for a Therapeutic Use Exemption (TUE) under the rules of their sport.

3 Contact ASADA to apply for a TUE. The contact details for ASADA are at the end of this chapter.

Advice for sports trainers and other coaching staff

As a sports trainer or a person on the coaching staff, you are in a position of trust, influence and respect. For this reason, you can be a valuable source of education for your athletes and have a direct impact on reducing drug use in your sport. You can do this by following the guidelines below.

■ Ensure non-medical personnel do not dispense or recommend any prescription medications to your athletes.

■ Ensure medications are used only as directed and that recommended doses are not exceeded.

■ Document the use of any medications by your athletes for future reference.

■ Clearly and effectively communicate your beliefs to your athletes. Your opinion will affect their decisions regarding drug use.

■ Provide only accurate and unexaggerated information about drug use. If you need more information, do some research or speak to a medical professional. Your athletes will rely on

a non-technical interpretation of information supplied by another medical professional.

■ Discourage the sharing of medications for what may appear to be similar complaints.

■ Discourage smoking.

■ Discourage binge drinking of alcohol and avoid rewarding athletes with alcohol. Be a role model in this regard.

■ Never administer or recommend any drugs to athletes. Refer them to a medical professional.

■ Be aware that many over-the-counter drugs may contain banned substances.

■ Advise your athletes to always tell their treating doctor that they are athletes subject to doping control under the rules of their sport.

Coaches, administrators, senior players, sports trainers, fitness instructors, teachers and parents play a very important role in creating a healthy sporting environment and influencing attitudes towards appropriate drug use.

Rules relating to drug use in sport change frequently. For example, on 1 January each year WADA releases an updated Prohibited List. For further information on safe drug and substance practices relevant to your sport, refer to the details below.

ASADA

ASADA is the organisation responsible for the implementation of the World Anti-Doping Code in Australia. It deters the use of banned doping practices in sport via education, testing, advocacy and coordination of Australia's anti-doping program. Athletes and support personnel should visit the ASADA website regularly for notifications of updates and changes.

ASADA has a single contact telephone number for all inquiries, including application for TUEs – 13000 ASADA (13000 27232).

Further information can be found on the ASADA website (www.asada.gov.au).

Other useful websites and resources

■ CleanEdge – Sports Medicine Australia's Anti-Doping and Body Image Program – www.cleanedge.com.au

■ World Anti Doping Agency – www.wada-ama.org

■ Australian Drug Information Network – www.adin.com.au

■ Australian Drug Foundation – www.adf.org.au

■ Alcohol and other Drugs Council of Australia – www.adca.org.au

Chapter Six

PRINCIPLES OF INJURY MANAGEMENT

LEARNING OUTCOMES

Identify the context and operations of a sports trainer in accordance with accepted principles of injury management.

1   Define and apply the DRSABCD principle for crisis management.
2   Define and apply the STOP principle.
3   Define and apply the TOTAPS principle.
4   Detail how to question injured athletes.
5   Describe the basic principles underlying assessment of an injury.

ASSESSMENT OF OUTCOMES

Underpinning knowledge

Oral or written questions may be asked relating to the principles and practices of injury management in a sporting context. You may also be asked to complete an online learning task related to the principles of injury management and submit copies of completed online tasks.

Practical demonstration

You may be asked to show the treatment of your athletes or manage medical documentation. You may be required to identify specific sporting injuries and use sports medicine equipment in the treatment of these injuries.

Scenario

You may be asked to perform one or more treatments of a range of sports-related injuries. You may also be asked to complete all necessary documents and complete a handover to other medical personnel.

Introduction

The primary role of the sports trainer is to prevent injury and improve safety in sport. However, the risk of injury always exists in the sporting environment so, in the absence of more qualified medical personnel, it is the responsibility of the sports trainer to appropriately assess and manage the situation, at least until more qualified help arrives. The sports trainer should calmly approach the situation and apply established procedures based on up-to-date medical knowledge. This chapter describes a set of injury management principles that can guide the sports trainer in the management of sports-related injuries. These principles can be applied regardless of the type or severity of the injury. It is assumed that the sports trainer has a high degree of first-aid proficiency, which is a prerequisite for all sports trainers.

The basic principles of injury management that sports trainers should be guided by are:

- Before acting, check for potential danger to yourself as well as to other athletes and bystanders. Continue to reassess the situation and ensure your continued safety as well as that of other athletes and bystanders.
- Rapidly assess the situation, including noting what has happened, how many athletes are involved and their general condition.
- Call for help as soon as it is possible and safe to do so.
- Assess the response of each athlete – unconscious athletes have priority of care.
- Unless the condition is minor, or there is imminent danger, do not move the athlete. If an athlete must be moved, immobilise suspected fractures beforehand if it is possible.
- If the accident was not witnessed, treat the athlete as if they have sustained a spinal injury and immobilise them appropriately.
- An unconscious person who is breathing should be placed on their side (lateral position) to avoid choking and should be moved, if necessary, in this same position.
- When carrying an athlete on a stretcher, ensure all movements are as smooth as possible and that the stretcher remains horizontal.
- Explain to the athlete everything that is being done and continue to reassure them to minimise fear and improve cooperation.

Chain of survival

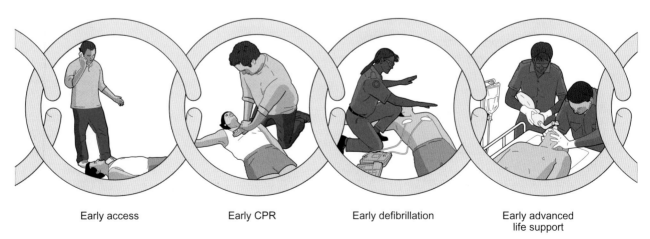

| Early access | Early CPR | Early defibrillation | Early advanced life support |

Figure 6.1 The chain of survival

The assessment and management of a collapsed or apparently unresponsive person is based on the concept of the 'chain of survival'. This is a series of linked actions that greatly increase a person's chance of survival and are usually defined as:

- Early access – call emergency services for help as soon as possible and get to the athlete to provide immediate assistance. This is sometimes referred to instead as early recognition.
- Early cardiopulmonary resuscitation (CPR) – effective CPR can maintain cardiac output and provide oxygen to the brain.
- Early defibrillation – defibrillation to restore normal heart function is applied as soon as possible.
- Early advanced life support – trained personnel, such as doctors or paramedics, apply interventions such as medication, artificial airways or ventilation.

For an athlete to have the best chance of survival, sports trainers must act quickly to assess the athlete's condition, seek medical assistance and begin resuscitation until more qualified help arrives. CPR greatly increases the chance of survival.

All athletes who have collapsed or require crisis management for any reason must be sent to hospital, even if they appear to have fully recovered.

DRSABCD principles

Basic life support (BLS) is emergency treatment to maintain life with little or no equipment. The guidelines for BLS in Australia are continually monitored and regularly updated by the Australian Resuscitation Council in line with the latest available medical research and scientific opinion. The current BLS guidelines are commonly referred to by the acronym DRSABCD. They are also often referred to as the CPR guidelines.

Regardless of the reason or circumstances leading to a person collapsing or becoming apparently unresponsive, the principles of DRSABCD apply to all first aid cases. They provide the starting point for sports trainers in their assessment and management of an athlete.

DRSABCD principles

D	Dangers?
R	Responsive?
S	Send for help
A	Open Airway
B	Normal Breathing?
C	Start CPR
D	Attach Defibrillator

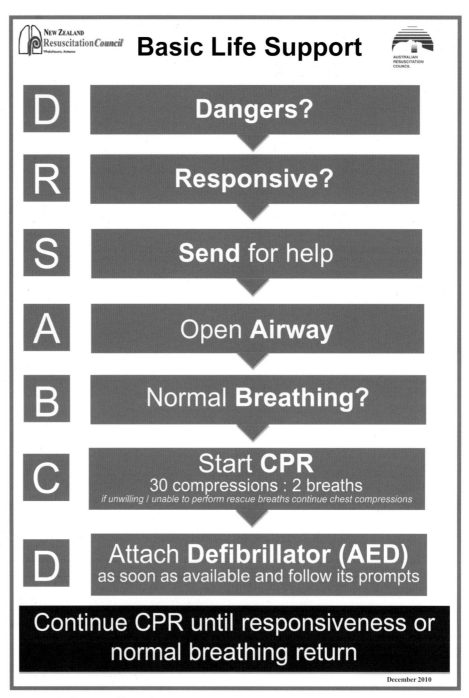

Figure 6.2 The Basic Life Support flow chart

Dangers?

Before attempting any further assessment or treatment, first check the area for danger to yourself, the athlete(s) and bystanders. As the rescuer, you should not put yourself in a situation where there is a risk of personal injury or death. You cannot help others if you add yourself to the casualty list by exposing yourself to danger.

Check the area around the site of the incident for anything that may cause further injury to the athlete or prevent you from helping them (e.g. electrical cables, sharp objects, dangerous wildlife etc). In a sporting situation, danger may be present in the form of other players, moving vehicles or other equipment. Always remember to check in all directions – 'look up, look down, look around' is a good principle to remember.

Move the athlete only if it is necessary to do so because of emerging danger that cannot be avoided or eliminated. If danger is present and the athlete cannot be attended to or removed safely, seek expert assistance, such as paramedics, and wait for them to arrive.

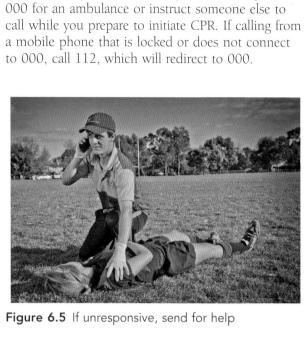

Figure 6.3 Check for danger

Responsive?

It is necessary to determine if the athlete is conscious or apparently unconscious. Gently squeeze the athlete's shoulders and use the COWS phrases to assess the athlete's response.

COWS phrases

C	**C**an you hear me?
O	**O**pen your eyes
W	**W**hat is your name?
S	**S**queeze my hand

While assessing whether they are responsive, be careful not to move the athlete's neck.

If the athlete is responsive, place them in the lateral position and continue to monitor them until help arrives. If they are not responsive, continue with the DRSABCD principles.

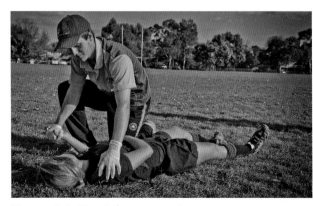

Figure 6.4 Check for responsiveness

Send for help

If there is no response, the person must be regarded as unconscious, so immediately send for help. Call 000 for an ambulance or instruct someone else to call while you prepare to initiate CPR. If calling from a mobile phone that is locked or does not connect to 000, call 112, which will redirect to 000.

Figure 6.5 If unresponsive, send for help

Open airway

Check that the airway is open and unobstructed by objects such as loose mouth guards, broken teeth, vomit etc. Do not remove mouth guards or dentures unless they are loose and interfering with the athlete's airway.

If foreign matter is present and it cannot be removed easily, it may be easier to roll the athlete into the lateral position first. However, remember that it is important to always suspect a spinal injury in an unconscious athlete, so ensure that a neutral alignment of the neck is maintained while moving them into the side lying position.

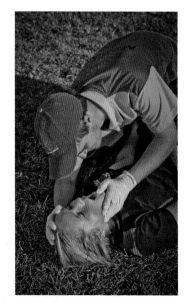

Figure 6.6 Check for an open airway

To maintain an open airway, pull the jaw forward (jaw thrust) while also minimising movement of the neck.

Breathing?

With the athlete lying on their side or back, check for breathing using the principles of 'look, listen and feel'.

- Look and feel – can you see or feel their chest rising and falling?
- Listen and feel – with your ear about 5 cm from the athlete's nose and mouth, listen for sounds of air entering and leaving the lungs. Can you feel their breath on your cheek?

If there is doubt about whether the athlete is breathing, assume they are not and commence CPR. Abnormal breathing should be considered as not breathing and is also an indication to start CPR.

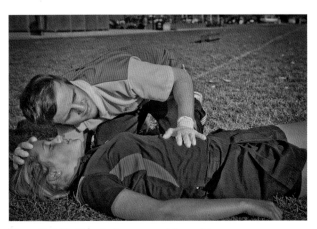

Figure 6.7 Check for normal breathing

Start CPR

If the athlete is not responsive and not breathing properly, external cardiac compressions should be started immediately, preferably in combination with mouth-to-mouth rescue breaths. The ratio of compressions should be 30 compressions to every 2 breaths (30:2) at an overall rate of 100 compressions per minute.

The rescuer's hands should be placed on the lower half of the sternum in the centre of the chest. The depth of compression should be one-third of the depth of the chest.

Rescue breaths should be delivered at approximately one second each while watching for the chest to rise. If the rescuer is unwilling or unable to perform rescue breaths, external cardiac compressions should continue uninterrupted.

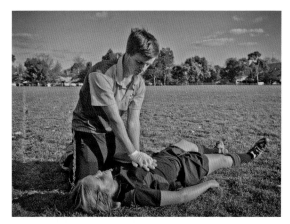

Figure 6.8 External cardiac compression

Attach a defibrillator (AED)

As soon as one is available, attach an automated external defibrillator (AED), turn it on and follow the prompts provided by the AED. Early defibrillation significantly improves the chance of survival. If the casualty has any form of heart rhythm disturbance, the AED can detect this and deliver a shock that might return the heart to a normal rhythm.

Continue CPR, including following prompts by the AED, until qualified personnel arrive or signs of life return.

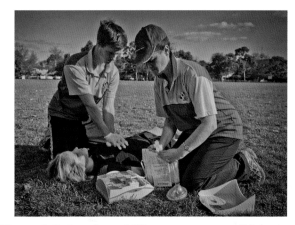

Figure 6.9 Attach an AED as soon as possible

AEDs are simple and safe to use and cannot harm a person, even if they are applied to someone with a normal pulse, as the AED will detect this and not deliver a shock. All sports clubs and venues should consider obtaining an AED and locating it where it can be readily accessed in the event of a medical emergency. Figure 6.11 shows the standard sign used in Australia that indicates the location of an AED.

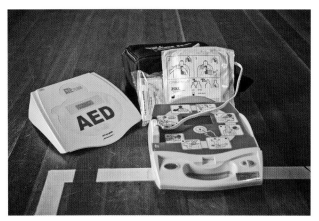

Figure 6.10 An automated defibrillator unit (AED)

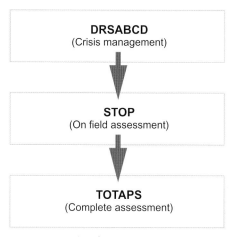

Figure 6.12 Principles for managing injured athletes

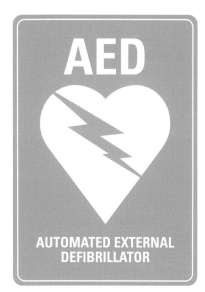

Figure 6.11 Standard sign indicating the location of an AED

Approach to the management of an injured athlete

Sports trainers should use a standardised approach to the assessment and management of an injured athlete. Once it is clear that the athlete's life is not in danger and that they are breathing normally after following the DRSABCD principles, the sports trainer can commence an assessment of what other assistance should be provided. The usual process following the application of the DRSABCD principles is to conduct a quick initial on-field assessment using the STOP principles and then, depending on the outcome of this assessment, continue to a more detailed assessment using the TOTAPS principles.

On-field assessment (STOP principles)

The STOP principles can be used to guide a fast on-field assessment. STOP is conducted after life-threatening problems have been managed using the DRSABCD principles and once it is clear that the athlete's life is not in immediate danger.

STOP principles

S	**S**top the athlete from moving or further participating. Stop the game if necessary
T	**T**alk to the injured athlete. (What happened? How did it happen? What did you feel? Where does it hurt?)
O	**O**bserve while talking to the athlete
P	**P**revent further injury

Depending on the outcome of the STOP assessment, the sports trainer should be able to decide if the athlete:

1 can remain on the field and continue to play, with or without further treatment

2 should remain on the field of play for further treatment due to the risk of further harm if they are moved

3 can be safely moved off the field for a more detailed assessment using the TOTAPS principles.

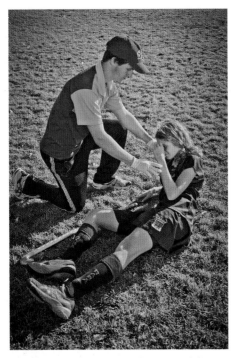

Figure 6.13 The STOP principle is used for on-field assessment

When using TOTAPS to assess an injury, the sports trainer is aiming to answer the following three questions:

1 Is there an injury present?
2 How severe is the injury – can the athlete continue playing or not?
3 Is it possible to determine the type of the injury (e.g. hard tissue or soft tissue)?

By answering these questions, the sports trainer can gain appropriate information to assist in deciding what immediate management is appropriate for this athlete:

1 whether the athlete requires further management or can continue to play
2 if further management is required, whether the athlete needs to go to hospital now or if they should be referred to a health professional for medical assessment and treatment either now or later.

TOTAPS can be used if there is more than one injury, or if there is more than one injured player, to determine which injuries should be treated first. Based on this assessment, available resources and personnel can be appropriately allocated.

While conducting the STOP assessment the sports trainer should look for signs of obvious injury such as bleeding, wounds, fractures, burns, swelling, bruising or any other type of observable deformity or signs. This secondary part of the assessment is conducted prior to moving the athlete or determining what treatment can or should be provided while still on the field of play.

Complete assessment (TOTAPS principles)

TOTAPS is a framework of questions and observations that is used to make a full assessment, usually off the field. This should occur only after DRSABCD and STOP have been completed.

TOTAPS is used as a guide to:
- specifically assess the injury
- implement appropriate injury management.

To make a detailed assessment the TOTAPS approach is used.

TALK

Talking to the athlete can provide useful information as to what happened during the current incident as well as any relevant previous history that might guide further management of their condition.

Some of the questions to ask the athlete include:
- What happened to cause the incident?
- What happened to the injured person during the incident?
- What is the problem now?
- Where does it hurt?
- Has a similar injury occurred before?

The answers to these questions may give the sports trainer guidance as to what sort of immediate management is most appropriate and can also be recorded on the injury report form. This can, in turn, assist those to whom the athlete is referred for further assessment and care.

As well as talking to the injured athlete, the sports trainer can also obtain information from other players, officials or spectators who saw the event.

In checking the history of the athlete, ask about:
- any previous injuries to this body part
- any previous injuries to the same part on the opposite side of the body
- any other recent injuries
- any other medical conditions they may have (e.g. diabetes or asthma).

Once the sports trainer has identified the location of the main problem, the next step can commence.

TOTAPS principles

T	Talk to the injured athlete
O	Observe the injured area
T	Touch the injured area
A	Active movement assessment
P	Passive movement assessment
S	Skills test

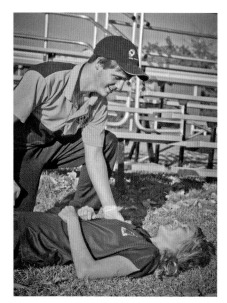

Figure 6.14 Talk (TOTAPS)

OBSERVE

To observe the injured area, compare the injured side to the uninjured side.

Look for:
- swelling
- deformity
- discolouration
- how the athlete is moving or holding the painful area.

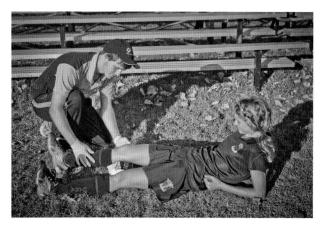

Figure 6.15 Observe (TOTAPS)

If an obvious injury or deformity is observed that requires immediate first aid treatment, such as an obvious fracture, appropriate first aid should now commence. If no obvious injury is observed, the sports trainer can then move on to the next component of TOTAPS, which is 'touch'.

TOUCH

Touch should only occur after the steps of talking and observing have occurred. Touch is undertaken to feel for a deformity that is not immediately visible by observation alone and also to pinpoint areas of tenderness.

Ask the athlete if you can examine the injured area and instruct them to tell you if it becomes too painful or if they want you to stop.

To complete the touch assessment:
- compare with the opposite side of the body
- begin touching away from the injury and slowly and gently move towards the injury site
- feel for tenderness, temperature and pain
- locate the exact site of pain
- assess if the site of the injury is hot and/or swollen
- check for any unusual lumps or bumps.

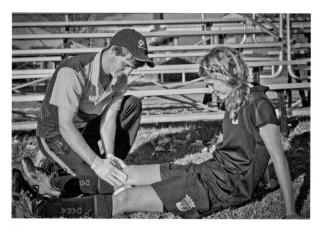

Figure 6.16 Touch (TOTAPS)

ACTIVE MOVEMENT

Active movement helps to determine if the athlete has any limitation of movement or hesitation due to pain or discomfort.

Complete the active movement assessment by asking the athlete to move the injured part through its normal range of movement, but only to the point of pain or discomfort. If necessary, demonstrate the desired movement. Observe the movement but do not touch or assist the athlete in any way. If movement is not obviously limited it may be useful to ask them to move the uninjured side for comparison.

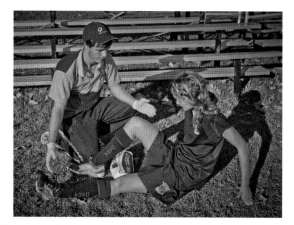

Figure 6.17 Active movement (TOTAPS)

To assess active movement, perform the following:

- Observe if there is a full or restricted range of motion.
- Observe if the athlete is 'guarding' by moving slowly or cautiously.
- Observe how the injured side moves compared to the uninjured side.
- Ask the athlete if there is pain when moving and, if so, when the pain occurs.
- If pain is present, ask the athlete to rate the pain on a scale of 0–10 where 0 is no pain at all and 10 is the worst pain imaginable.
- If there is pain or limitation of movement, stop the assessment at that point and begin management of the injury.
- If the athlete does not complain of pain, continue onto assessment of passive movement.

PASSIVE MOVEMENT

Passive movement assessment is conducted by the sports trainer to identify whether the movement observed during assessment of active movement is full and unrestricted compared to the full available range of movement.

To assess passive movement, perform the following:

- Ask first if the athlete is agreeable to you moving the injured area.
- Gently move the affected body part through the full range of movement.
- Compare the range of movement between the injured and uninjured sides.
- Ask if pain occurs during the movement and, if so, at what point or range of movement.

The sports trainer should carefully move the joint through its normal range of movement if possible, but only to the point of pain or restriction if this occurs. If there is pain, do not push the injured area past that point: instead, stop the assessment and begin management.

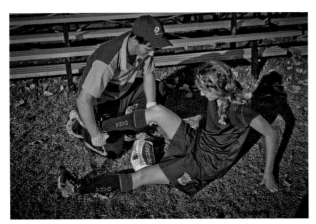

Figure 6.18 Passive movement (TOTAPS)

SKILLS TEST

A skills test can be undertaken if the athlete can move the injured joint through its full range of movement without pain. The skills test is used to determine if the athlete is able to return to play or instead should be referred for further assessment or care. A skills test progressively takes the athlete through relevant sports specific skills, from easy to more difficult, to determine if they can safely and effectively perform the activities required of them on the field of play.

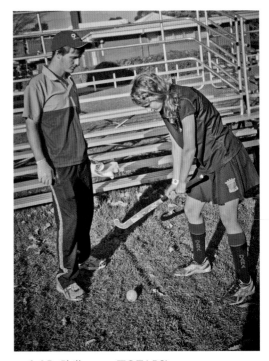

Figure 6.19 Skills test (TOTAPS)

If using any of these skills causes pain or the athlete is unable to complete them, they should not return to activity and appropriate management should be commenced or continued. For example, a suitable progression of skills test for a footballer who has sustained a suspected ankle injury might start with standing, followed by walking, walking in a circle or figure of eight, jogging, running, jumping, sidestepping and kicking a ball with either foot.

If pain occurs during the assessment process, the RICER and NO HARM principles can be used to guide further management of the athlete's injury. These are discussed in Chapter 7.

Handover to other medical personnel

SAMPLE principles

If an ambulance has been called, the sports trainer should stay with the athlete, reassure them and continue to assess them using the DRSABCD and STOP principles until the athlete can be handed over to the ambulance officers/paramedics.

All athletes treated by a sports trainer should be referred further for the appropriate medical care with continuing or follow-up treatment. When handing an athlete over to paramedics or when referring an athlete to a health professional, sports trainers can use the SAMPLE principles to provide a summary of information relating to the athlete's condition that may be helpful.

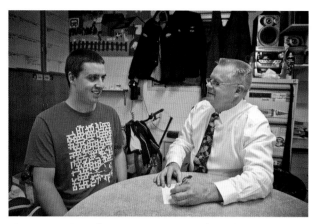

Figure 6.20 Follow-up assessment by a health professional

SAMPLE principles

S	**S**igns and symptoms – what signs and symptoms does the athlete currently have?
A	**A**llergies – does the athlete have any known allergies to medication, food, insects etc?
M	**M**edication – what medications is the athlete currently taking, if any?
P	**P**ast medical record – has a similar injury occurred in the past?
L	**L**ast meal – when did the athlete last eat and drink? What did they have?
E	**E**vent – what happened leading up to the incident?

Chapter Seven

COMMON SPORTING ILLNESSES AND INJURIES

LEARNING OUTCOMES

Demonstrate care and management of athletes suffering from sporting-related injuries and illnesses.

1. Define and apply the RICER and NO HARM principles.
2. Recognise and manage athletes with hard and soft tissue injuries.
3. Recognise and manage head and spinal injuries.
4. Recognise and manage trunk injuries.
5. Recognise and manage upper limb injuries.
6. Recognise and manage lower limb injuries.
7. Recognise and manage heat and cold injuries and illness.
8. Recognise and manage signs and symptoms of shock.
9. Recognise and manage serious bleeding.
10. Apply wound management principles appropriate to sport.

ASSESSMENT OF OUTCOMES

Underpinning knowledge

Oral or written questions may be asked relating to the principles and practices of injury and illness management in a sporting context. You may also be asked to complete an online learning task related to principles of injury management and submit copies of completed online tasks.

Practical demonstration

You may be asked to show treatment of your athletes or manage medical documentation. You may be required to identify specific sporting injuries and use sports medicine equipment in the treatment of these injuries.

Scenario

You may be asked to perform one or more treatments for a range of sports-related injuries. You may also be asked to complete all necessary documents and complete a handover to other medical personnel.

Introduction

This chapter examines the management of some of the more common injuries and medical conditions that can occur in sport, particularly those that are more serious and that require rapid, correct care. This assumes competence in first aid and builds on the competencies in the Apply First Aid course but with a sports focus.

Due to the nature and demands of sport and exercise, the human body can sustain a range of injuries or be exposed to certain types of medical conditions. Although the possibility of sports-related injuries and medical conditions represents an ongoing risk to participants, this must be contrasted with the proven health benefits of sport and physical activity, especially compared to health conditions and illnesses that are likely to occur with inactivity or sedentary behaviour. These health benefits include improvement in nearly all aspects of human health, including cardiovascular, skeletal and muscular health as well as psychological and emotional wellbeing.

Shock

Shock is a term used to describe the loss of effective circulation. As a result of inadequate circulation the oxygen supplied to the body's tissues is less than required for normal function. This can lead to the shutdown and death of body tissues, including vital organs such as the brain, lungs and heart. Urgent medical attention is necessary in all cases of shock or suspected shock to prevent the risk of serious permanent tissue damage or the death of the affected person.

Causes of shock

Shock can occur in conjunction with any injury or medical condition but is most commonly associated with:

- blood loss as a result of external or internal bleeding
- burns
- fluid loss from severe diarrhoea, vomiting, sweating or dehydration
- cardiac emergencies
- brain or spinal cord injury
- severe infections
- allergic reactions
- major or multiple fractures
- major trauma.

Signs of shock

- Reduced level of consciousness
- Rapid, weak pulse
- Rapid breathing
- Vomiting
- Pale, cold or clammy skin

All these signs usually appear within the first hour of an injury.

Symptoms of shock

- Faintness or dizziness
- Trembling or weakness in the arms and legs
- Enlarged (dilated) pupils
- Nausea
- Restlessness or anxiety
- Confusion

Management of shock

For athletes with severe injuries, illness or infection, shock should be anticipated as early intervention and appropriate care may prevent shock from developing. Management of shock includes:

- If any signs or symptoms of shock are present, seek medical help urgently.
- If the athlete is apparently unresponsive, commence the DRSABCD principles.
- Lay the athlete on their back in a horizontal position to maintain circulation to the trunk. Do not elevate the head.
- If a head or spinal injury is not suspected, raise the athlete's legs but keep the head level with the heart.
- Loosen any tight clothing or protective equipment.
- Protect the athlete from extremes of temperature.
- Moisten the athlete's lips, but do not give drinks or food.
- Continue to monitor the athlete closely as they may deteriorate rapidly.

Serious bleeding

The standard procedure for treating an athlete with serious life-threatening bleeding is:

- Treat the athlete for shock.
- Send for medical help.
- Apply and maintain direct pressure to control bleeding. Pressure is applied using gloved fingers or the heel of the hand in conjunction with sterile or clean compress pads, bandages or towels.
- If bleeding is heavy or a dressing is not available, grasp the sides of the wound and press them firmly together.
- If bleeding persists, do not remove the dressing. Apply further pads and bandaging.
- In the case of bleeding from a limb, elevate the injured part while supporting any suspected fracture.
- Do not try to clean major bleeding as stopping the bleeding using direct pressure is critical.
- Apply oxygen therapy when it is available and qualified personnel are present.
- Arterial tourniquets are not recommended.

Hard tissue injuries

Hard tissue injuries are injuries that affect the bones and include fractures of actual bones as well as dislocations and subluxations of the joints between bones. If in doubt as to whether a fracture or dislocation is present, a hard tissue injury should be treated as a fracture.

Fractures

A fracture is an injury where bone tissue loses its normal structure, usually as a result of direct or indirect trauma. There are many different types of fractures; they can be classified according to the type of damage to the bone (e.g.complete/incomplete, displaced/undisplaced) as well as whether the fractured bone penetrates the skin and causes an open wound (open fracture/closed fracture – see Figure 7.1). Fractures can also be classified according to the cause, such as stress fractures, which commonly occur in sport because of overuse or biomechanical problems the athlete might have.

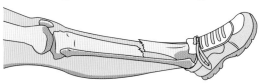

Open fracture of the tibia

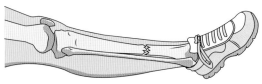

Closed fracture of the tibia

Figure 7.1 Fractures of the tibia

Both open and closed fractures have the potential to cause serious injury to internal body structures. Although many fractures are not immediately life threatening, fractures can cause shock and major internal and external bleeding.

Fractures usually present with:
- the occurrence of a forceful episode
- falling
- being hit by an object or opponent
- possible deformity or swelling
- localised tenderness, and/or a deep aching pain.

SIGNS OF A FRACTURE
- Deformity – the affected part is changed in shape
- Bone protruding from an open wound
- Localised swelling
- Movement in a limb occurring other than at a joint
- Loss of normal movement or function
- Signs of shock

SYMPTOMS OF A FRACTURE
- Pain and tenderness at the site
- The sound of a snap or pop at the time of injury
- Feeling/sound of bone ends grating
- Tingling or numbness
- Symptoms of shock

MANAGEMENT OF FRACTURES
Acute management of fractures depends on the location of the injury and the type of fracture; however, for the purposes of providing immediate treatment, the following steps apply to most fractures.
- Follow DRSABCD principles as appropriate.
- If the athlete is conscious, reassure them and advise them not to move.
- Call for an ambulance or medical assistance.
- Control bleeding if there is an open wound and cover it with a sterile dressing to reduce infection.
- Check that circulation is present distal to the fracture. If not, call for urgent medical aid.
- If the athlete needs to be moved, immobilise the area of the suspected fracture first.
- Immobilise the injured limb in the position you found it.
- Be sure to immobilise the area above and below the fracture.
- If the fracture needs to be splinted, the splint must be long enough to extend past the joints

above and below the fracture site as well as wide enough to support the fracture site.

- Check the athlete for other injuries and treat appropriately.
- Apply ice packs or cold compresses, if possible, for up to 20 minutes if pain permits. Reapply ice every 2 hours if necessary. Do not apply ice to open fractures.
- Assess for shock and treat as required.

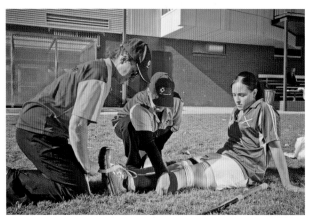

Figure 7.2 Splinting a suspected fracture

MANAGEMENT OF SKULL FRACTURES

Skull fractures may be characterised by:
- watery blood from the nose or ears
- swelling or a bump on the skull
- depression in the skull
- bleeding from the scalp.

Management of skull fractures includes the following steps:
- Rest and prevent the athlete from sustaining possible further harm.
- Reassure the athlete.
- Place the athlete in a position of comfort if possible.
- Suspect spinal injury and treat accordingly.

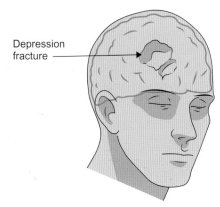

Depression fracture

Figure 7.3 Skull fracture

MANAGEMENT OF UPPER AND LOWER ARM FRACTURES

- Control bleeding if there is an open wound and cover it with a sterile dressing to reduce infection. Apply padding around any protruding bones.
- For lower arm fractures, apply a splint from the elbow to the hand to immobilise the fracture. Support the fracture using a broad arm sling.
- If the suspected fracture involves the elbow or is very close to it, do not move the elbow. Support and immobilise the arm in the position you found it.
- For upper arm fractures, place a pad between the arm and the chest and apply an elevated arm sling to immobilise the arm.
- Check that circulation is present beyond the fracture. If not, call for urgent medical aid.
- Check the athlete for other injuries and treat appropriately.

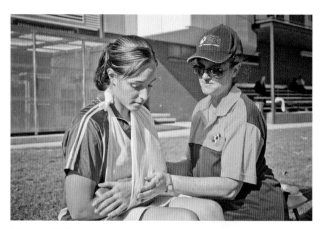

Figure 7.4 Splint and sling for a suspected lower arm fracture

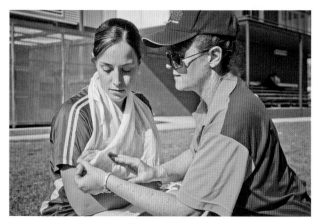

Figure 7.5 Checking for circulation

MANAGEMENT OF UPPER AND LOWER LEG FRACTURES

- Control bleeding if there is an open wound and cover it with a sterile dressing to reduce infection. Apply padding around protruding bones.

- The uninjured leg may be used as a splint for upper and lower leg fractures. Place a pad or splinting material between the legs, bring the uninjured leg to the injured leg and tie the legs together with bandages above and below the suspected fracture. Tie off on the uninjured side.
- If the ground is supporting the limb adequately there may be no need to splint it to the other limb.
- Check that circulation is present beyond the fracture. If not, call for urgent medical aid.
- Check the athlete for other injuries and treat appropriately.

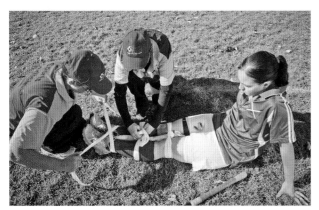

Figure 7.6 Splinting for a suspected lower limb fracture

MANAGEMENT OF HIP FRACTURES

- Control bleeding if there is an open wound and cover it with a sterile dressing to prevent infection. Apply padding around protruding bones.
- The uninjured leg may be used as a splint for hip fractures. Place a pad between the legs, bring the uninjured leg to the injured leg and tie the legs together with triangular bandages above and below the fracture, at the knees and at the ankles/feet. Tie off on the uninjured side.
- Do not move the athlete unless they are in life-threatening danger. If they must be moved, immobilise them on a spinal board or similar hard surface.
- Check for signs of circulation distal to the fracture site.
- Monitor vital signs and treat for shock.

MANAGEMENT OF PELVIC FRACTURES

- Control bleeding if there is an open wound and cover it with a sterile dressing to prevent

infection. Apply padding around protruding bones.

- Place the legs and feet in a position of comfort.
- Discourage the athlete from urinating.
- Monitor vital signs and treat for shock.
- Do not move the athlete unless they are in life-threatening danger. If they must be moved, immobilise them on a spinal board or similar hard surface.

MANAGEMENT OF RIB FRACTURES

- Ensure the athlete is in a comfortable position. If possible, allow them to find their own position of comfort. A half-sitting position resting the affected side on a pillow or cushion is ideal.
- Encourage shallow breathing to reduce pain.
- Apply padding over the affected ribs.
- Place the arm that is on the same side as the injury over the pad.
- Secure the pad with broad bandages over the arm and around the body, tying them off on the non-injured side.
- Immobilise the arm using an appropriate sling.
- Seek medical assistance.
- Be aware that breathing difficulties may be associated with rib fractures.

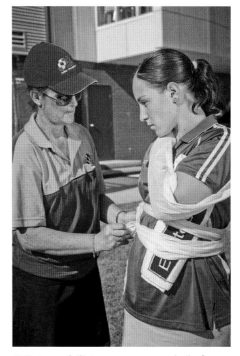

Figure 7.7 Immobilising a suspected rib fracture

Hard tissue injuries in young athletes

The principles of injury assessment and management of fractures in children and young people are the same as for adults. However, it is important to be aware of possible fractures or dislocations in younger athletes as fractures may occur through the growth plate region (epiphysis) of the bone. Incorrectly treated fractures of the growth plate can cause an interruption in the growth of the bone, which can lead to permanent disabilities.

Dislocations

A dislocation is an injury in which a bone is moved out of its normal position within a joint with another bone. The most common examples in sport are dislocations of the fingers and the shoulder joint. Dislocations often cause considerable pain and muscle spasm. They also can cause damage to the joint capsule and surrounding ligaments and may affect surrounding nerves and muscles. It is often difficult for a sports trainer to tell the difference between a dislocation and a fracture or even a joint sprain. If in doubt, treatment should be given as though for a suspected fracture. Dislocations may also be associated with fractures of bones in or near the affected joint so, for all dislocations, a follow-up X-ray should be arranged. This is true whether or not the dislocated joint has been relocated to its usual position.

SIGNS OF A DISLOCATION
- Loss of function
- Swelling at the site
- Deformity

SYMPTOMS OF A DISLOCATION
- Pain and tenderness at the site of the injury

MANAGEMENT OF A DISLOCATION
- Do not attempt to reposition the dislocated joint.
- Prevent movement occurring at the site of the dislocation to reduce the risk of further tissue damage.
- Immobilise the injured limb in the position you found it.
- Gently apply a splint and sling. Be sure to immobilise the area above and below the injured joint.
- Check for signs of circulation below the dislocation.
- If possible, apply ice packs or cold compresses for up to 20 minutes at a time to relieve pain. Reapply if necessary.
- Treat for shock where appropriate.

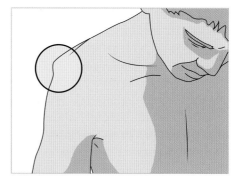

Figure 7.8 Right anterior shoulder dislocation demonstrating loss of normal shoulder contour

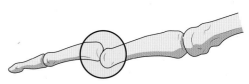

Figure 7.9 Dislocation of an interphalangeal joint of the finger

RULES FOR MANAGING DISLOCATIONS
- Remember that the sports trainer should not attempt to relocate or reduce the dislocation of any joint.
- For all dislocations a referral for follow-up medical assessment is essential.
- A follow-up X-ray should be arranged for all dislocations to check for associated fractures.
- Do not give the athlete anything to eat or drink.

Subluxation

Subluxations are incomplete dislocations. As with dislocations, subluxations may cause damage to the joint capsule and surrounding ligaments. Treat as for a dislocation.

Soft tissue injuries

Soft tissue injuries involve tissues other than bone. With respect to musculoskeletal injuries, they include sprains of ligament tissue and strains of muscle tissue. If there is doubt about the severity of the injury and whether it involves soft or hard tissue, treat it as a fracture.

Soft tissue includes:
- Muscle – muscles consist of cells with a specific function, namely to contract to produce movement of the body. They are usually attached to bones by tendons. Muscles have an extensive blood supply and consequently may bleed heavily when injured.

The common injuries that occur to muscle tissue are strains and contusions/bruises.

- Tendons – tendons are tough bands of slightly elastic connective tissue that connect muscle to bone. Tendons relay the force the muscle produces to the bones to cause movement. Common injuries to tendons include strains or complete tears (rupture) and inflammation or degeneration of the tendon (tendinopathy).
- Ligaments – ligaments are strong bands of fibrous tissue that attach to adjacent bones in joints. They enhance the stability of the joint. An injured ligament is called a sprain.
- The joint capsule – this is the thin ligamentous tissue that surrounds joints and produces the lubricating synovial fluid found in joints. These tissues can also be injured with a joint strain, dislocation or subluxation.
- Skin and fatty tissue – an injury to any of these tissues is classified as a soft tissue injury.

Organs such as the brain, lungs or kidneys, although soft in nature, are not included in the definition of soft tissues.

Some soft tissue injuries may have a clear history of a particular cause or incident, whereas for others this will be unclear. Regardless of the cause, all soft tissue injuries can be managed using the **RICER** and **NO HARM** principles that are discussed later in this chapter.

Strains

A strain is a soft tissue injury involving muscle tissue and is usually caused by overstretching of the muscle. Strains vary from minor to major depending on the amount of muscle tissue that is damaged. A full-thickness tear of a muscle is often referred to as a complete muscle rupture; these ruptures may require surgical repair.

SIGNS OF A STRAIN

- Swelling
- Possible discolouration and bruising
- Loss of muscle strength

SYMPTOMS OF A STRAIN

- Pain on movement, especially where it involves resisted muscle contractions or stretching of the injured muscle

Sprains

Sprains occur when the ligaments that connect bones within a joint are forcibly stretched beyond their normal range, leading to stretching or tearing. Sprains vary from minor to major depending on the amount of ligament tissue that is damaged. A full-thickness tear of a ligament is often referred to as a complete ligament rupture; these usually require

prolonged immobilisation or surgery to repair or reattach the separated ends of the ligament.

SIGNS AND SYMPTOMS OF A SPRAIN

- Swelling
- Possible bruising or discolouration
- Pain on joint movement

Contusions

A contusion or bruise is a soft tissue injury affecting muscle tissue and blood vessels that bleed into the muscle. Contusions are usually caused by blunt trauma to the area. They usually respond well to **RICER** treatment. Gentle exercise or movement can usually be started within a few hours after the injury.

SIGNS OF A CONTUSION

- Swelling
- Discolouration

SYMPTOMS OF A CONTUSION

- Pain or tenderness at the site of the injury
- Muscle weakness or inhibition

Process of injury and repair in soft tissue injuries

As soft tissue injuries are the most prevalent injuries encountered in athletes it is useful for a sports trainer to have an understanding of the injury and repair process. A sports trainer will frequently have to explain this process to injured athletes in order to ensure adherence to the correct management of the injury.

There are eight stages in the process of injury and repair:

1. Initial tissue damage
2. Capillary bleeding
3. Clot formation
4. Tissue swelling
5. Secondary tissue damage
6. Removal of the blood clot and tissue swelling
7. Healing of the tissue
8. Regaining function

INITIAL TISSUE DAMAGE

When an injury occurs, there will be some degree of initial or primary tissue damage, such as tearing or compression of the tissue. Any subsequent excessive movement may increase the tissue damage and further delay recovery.

CAPILLARY BLEEDING

Soft tissues have a blood supply to provide them with the constant supply of oxygen and nutrients that are required by them for normal function. When soft tissue is damaged, the capillaries within that tissue are also damaged, resulting in bleeding at the injury site. The degree of capillary bleeding is dependent upon the type of tissue damaged and the extent of the damage. This capillary bleeding may continue for up to 24–72 hours, depending on the severity of the injury, movement after the injury and initial injury care. Some tissues will bleed more than others (e.g. muscle tissue will usually bleed significantly due to its profuse blood supply whereas tendons will bleed less because of their limited blood supply).

CLOT FORMATION

The blood lost within the damaged tissue will eventually clot. If the clot is disturbed, such as by movement, the bleeding will continue. The main aim in the management of soft tissue injuries is to restrict tissue damage and minimise capillary bleeding and thereby keep the blood clot to a minimum size.

SECONDARY TISSUE DAMAGE

Additional or secondary tissue damage may be caused by:

- movement, which may lead to the tearing of more tissue or cause more bleeding damage
- damaged capillaries that continue to bleed, hence causing some cells in the damaged tissue to not receive their required blood supply, thereby leading to further damage
- tissue swelling, which can compress the small blood vessels in the area and reduce circulation to the damaged area.

INFLAMMATION

Inflammation is a normal part of the healing process. Following an injury the inflammatory process occurs, resulting in increases in local tissue temperature, fluid and chemicals that help the body to clear damaged tissue and to initiate the healing process. Inflammation can also be associated with a temporary increase in localised pain.

HEALING OF TISSUE

Healing of the damaged tissue commences while the blood clot and associated tissue inflammation or swelling are being removed. Fibrous scar tissue can replace the damaged tissue. This scar tissue can reduce the length and elasticity of damaged tissue. Reducing excessive swelling, guided exercises and gentle stretching of the injured part while the scar tissue is being created can help to retain the tissue length. This increases the flexibility of the damaged tissues and therefore helps to reduce the risk of future injury.

REGAINING FUNCTION

Regaining the function of the injured area begins as the blood clot and tissue swelling are being removed and the new tissue is being laid down. The goal for the athlete and sports trainer is to restore all function to at least the pre-injury condition, not just to

alleviate pain. Different rehabilitation routines are used for different injuries. Guidance from a health professional on what sort of rehabilitation strategies and exercises should be used is strongly advised.

Management of soft tissue injuries

RICER PRINCIPLE

RICER is a basic treatment for acute soft tissue injuries and should be used by the sports trainer in the first 48–72 hours of injury. Prompt management of soft tissue injuries using RICER controls swelling immediately after the injury. RICER aims to minimise bleeding, swelling and further tissue damage. This, in turn, minimises creation of scar tissue in the damaged area, which improves the chance of achieving full recovery and prevents the likelihood of re-injury.

RICER stands for:

- **R**est
- **I**ce
- **C**ompression
- **E**levation
- **R**eferral

Rest

Have the injured athlete sit or lie down with the injured part supported carefully to prevent further injury. Do not allow the athlete to move the injured area excessively.

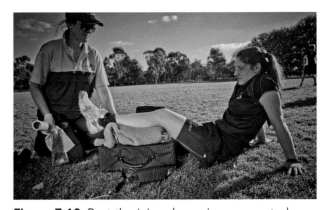

Figure 7.10 Rest the injured area in a supported position

Ice

Use ice or a cold pack to cool the affected area. A polythene bag filled with ice pieces and water is ideal. Wrap this in a damp cloth and place it on the injured site. Apply ice packs (covered by a towel or clothing to avoid burning of the skin) or cold compresses for 20 minutes every 2 hours for the first 48–72 hours following an injury.

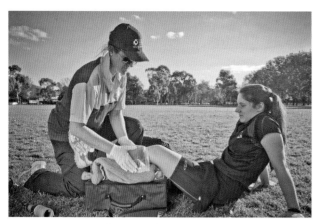

Figure 7.11 Apply ice and elevate the injured area above the heart

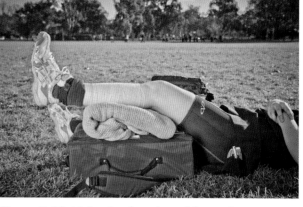

Figure 7.13 Maintain elevation while resting

Compression

Wrap a compression bandage around the injured area. This will help to support it and reduce movement and swelling at the site of injury. If using an ice pack, apply the compression bandaging over the ice pack or place the ice on top of the compression bandage. Check circulation is present beyond the bandage to ensure it is not too tight and also check the colour, warmth, movement and sensation in the area distal to the compression bandage.

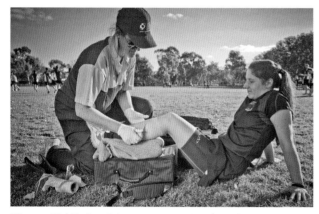

Figure 7.12 Applying compression bandaging

Elevation

If possible, raise the injured area above the level of the athlete's heart. This will reduce blood flow to the injured area, which in turn can reduce bleeding, swelling and pain. Support the elevated part with pillows, towels, slings etc.

Referral

Refer the injured athlete to an appropriate health care professional for a definitive diagnosis and appropriate continuing management. Provide the health professional with a written or verbal summary of the incident, including your observations and any treatment given, using the SAMPLE principle described in Chapter 6 or alternatively provide them with a copy of the injury report form.

NO HARM PRINCIPLE

The 'NO HARM principle' is the advice a sports trainer gives to any athlete who may have suffered a soft tissue injury to avoid making the injury worse. Advise the athlete to avoid the following for the first 48–72 hours.

Heat

Any type of heat will increase blood supply to the area, which can subsequently increase bleeding. Avoid heat packs or heat rubs and prolonged submersion of the injured part in hot showers, baths or saunas.

Alcohol

Consuming alcohol may increase bleeding and swelling. Alcohol causes blood vessels to dilate, which can increase bleeding in the injured area.

Running

Running or vigorous exercise of any sort, especially if that involves the injured part, may aggravate and worsen the injury if started too soon. Exercise and physical activity should be re-introduced gradually, and only without the presence of pain, following a diagnosis and recommendation by an appropriate health professional.

Massage

Massage in the early stages following injury can increase damage to already injured tissues and further increase swelling and bleeding within and around the injured structures. Vigorous massage of acute muscle contusions can lead to serious complications. Massage should only be started after risk factors have been excluded by a health professional.

Diagnosis by a qualified health professional should occur 48–72 hours after an injury. Arrange for a consultation with an appropriate medical or health professional, preferably one who has experience with sporting injuries, as soon as possible after the injury has occurred. With serious injuries, your referral would be an immediate call for an emergency medical service.

If the sports trainer applies the **RICER** and **NO HARM** principles correctly and early, the athlete is more likely to achieve as quick a return to sport as possible without additional complications arising from incorrect or delayed treatment. Minimising swelling and further tissue damage also assists health professionals involved in ongoing care by improving their ability to make an accurate early diagnosis without the distractions or masking of the actual injury by either excessive swelling or secondary complications and symptoms caused by incorrect treatment. Excessive swelling can also lead to a delay in the commencement of appropriate treatment and rehabilitation, which will add to the time before the athlete can return to sport.

Medications available for management of soft tissue injuries

Sports trainers should not recommend any type of medication to an athlete with a soft tissue injury. Although non-steroidal anti-inflammatory drugs (NSAIDs) have in the past been commonly used for treating acute soft tissue injuries, recent research has not found any convincing evidence as to their effectiveness, and they can cause side effects and complications in some people.

A doctor should be consulted for advice as to whether any type of medication may assist with the management of an athlete's soft tissue injuries.

TOPICAL NSAIDS

Topical NSAIDs are non-steroidal anti-inflammatory drugs that are applied to the injured area via a lotion, cream or spray. A sports trainer may apply this medication but only with the athlete's consent and following a doctor's recommendation. Ensure the athlete follows the directions on the packaging and does not exceed the recommended dose.

ORAL NSAIDS

Oral NSAIDs are non-steroidal anti-inflammatory drugs delivered in the form of a tablet, capsule or liquid. Many oral NSAIDs require a doctor's prescription. Unless medical advice has been obtained, NSAIDs should not be administered by a sports trainer due to possible contraindications or side effects they might cause.

Potential side effects from the use of anti-inflammatory drugs include dizziness, nausea and diarrhoea. Anti-inflammatory drugs can cause major problems for some people, especially those with preexisting gastrointestinal conditions, so a doctor should be consulted prior to taking these medications.

Overuse injuries

Overuse injuries occur as a result of an ongoing or constantly reapplied load that exceeds the body's capacity to recover from or repair, which eventually leads to tissue damage, usually involving bones, joint structures, tendons, muscles or a combination of these. There are many different types of overuse injuries in sport, some of which are specific to a particular sport or to the position played in that sport, and they arise because of the frequency with which a certain type of activity is performed. They all occur because of an abnormal load being placed on normal tissue.

These injuries can occur in athletes of all ages although some occur more frequently in children and adolescents, whereas others are more common in older athletes. Many sports-related overuse injuries

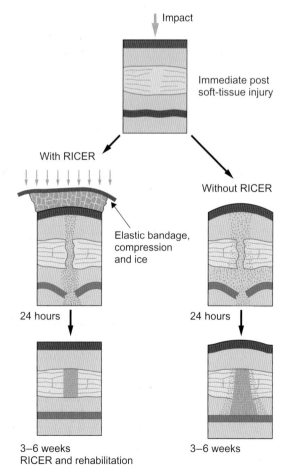

Figure 7.14 The importance of RICER

occur at or near the insertion point of tendons onto bone, including some of the common overuse injuries discussed below.

'Tennis elbow' (lateral epicondylitis)

Lateral epicondylitis is commonly known as tennis elbow, although it can occur as well in other sports and activities that involve a combination of both gripping and impact. It is an overuse injury affecting the outside or lateral aspect of the elbow. It usually occurs because of a repetitive or excessive load on the extensor tendons of the forearm that, in turn, transmits force to the muscles and tendons that attach to the bone on the outer lower part of the humerus (the lateral epicondyle).

In tennis, lateral epicondylagia is often associated with:

- an incorrect racquet grip size and/or a racquet that does not cushion impact well
- a one-handed backhand with poor technique, especially if the ball is hit with the front of the shoulder upwards causing excessive power generation by the forearm muscles
- a late forehand swing preparation with resulting wrist snap to bring the racquet head perpendicular to the ball
- a serving action with a wrist snap that increases the stress on the already taut extensor tendons.

'Golfer's elbow' (medial epicondylitis)

Medial epicondylitis or golfer's elbow is similar to lateral epicondylitis except it involves the inside (medial) part of the elbow. This overuse injury characteristically occurs with activities that involve wrist flexor activity and pronation, such as in golf, but can also occur in other sports including tennis. Medial epicondylitis can result from:

- late forehand biomechanics in tennis where the player quickly snaps the wrist to bring the racquet head forward
- the 'back-scratch' or cocking phase when serving, which places stress on the medial tissues of the elbow
- a golf swing where the club head is thrown down at the ball with the back arm rather than pulling the club through with the front arm and trunk
- improper pulling technique with certain swim strokes, especially the backstroke (also referred to as 'swimmer's elbow').

'Runner's knee'

Runner's knee is a term that can refer to a number of overuse conditions that commonly can cause pain around the front of the knee (patellofemoral pain) or the lateral part of the knee, as occurs in iliotibial band (ITB) syndrome.

Some of these conditions occur as a result of poor biomechanics, poor alignment of structures in and around the joint or weakness or tightness of the supporting and propulsive muscles. As well as biomechanical problems immediately around the knee, overuse injuries of the knee can also often be caused by foot, hip or pelvic problems or a combination of these.

'Shin splints' (medial tibial stress syndrome)

Shin splints is a non-specific general term that refers to exercise-related pain in the lower leg. It is common in many running-based sports, but also occurs commonly in dancers and people in the military. Shin splints are characterised by pain in the lower leg usually felt along the front and/or inside of the tibia. It may be painful to touch and varies in intensity according to activity and the stage of the injury.

As a result of repetitive strain, muscles attached to the tibia can cause inflammation, initially of the thin layer of tissue that covers the bone (periosteum). In time this can progress to a breakdown of the underlying bone, in other words a stress fracture.

Factors that might contribute to shin pain include:

- weakness or tightness of the lower leg muscles that control foot and ankle movement
- training errors, including a sudden increase in intensity, volume or duration of exercise or running on hard surfaces
- unsuitable, unsupportive or worn footwear
- biomechanical factors such as excessive pronation or excessive curvature of the tibia.

All of these injuries need to be referred to a qualified health practitioner for a definitive diagnosis. A sports trainer can assist by identifying the risk factors early and adjusting training programs where necessary.

Overuse injuries and young athletes

There are a number of possible hard and soft tissue injuries that can occur during growth periods in children and adolescents. These injuries often occur at or near:

1 growth plates in the bone
2 the insertion point of tendons into bones.

A combination of the rapid gain in bone length and the relative softness of these sites in children and adolescents can lead to strain, separation or detachment of bone or soft tissue.

There are many different types of conditions that fall into this broad category and, although they are often dismissed as 'growing pains', these can be serious conditions that must be assessed and managed by an appropriate health professional. Part of the management of growth-related musculoskeletal conditions usually involves specific recommendations as to the type and amount of exercise and training the young athlete should do. Sports trainers have an important role in ensuring young athletes follow recommendations from health professionals and that they warm up fully and do not overtrain.

Spinal injuries

Injuries to the head and spine can occur in sport, particularly contact sports, collision sports and those that have a risk of falls. The head and spine can be damaged through contact with another body, object or the environment. Injury to the head and spine can also occur as a result of indirect transmission of force due to acceleration/deceleration forces when the head movement stops or starts suddenly. Due to the important structures located in these areas, it is important that the sports trainer is able to assess these injuries and implement the appropriate initial management and subsequent referral.

Most spinal injuries occur in either the cervical or the lumbar regions of the spine. The two mechanisms operating in the majority of serious spinal injuries in sport are:

1 vertical compression
2 flexion with rotation.

The severity of spinal injuries is impossible to determine without appropriate medical imaging such as X-ray, CT or MRI scans; therefore, sports trainers need to refer all suspected spinal injury cases for further medical assessment and assistance.

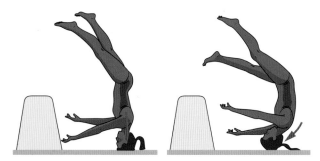

Figure 7.15 Vertical compression and forced flexion of the neck

Signs of spinal injury

- Breathing difficulties
- Profuse bleeding from the head or abrasions or bruising to the forehead
- Dilation or unequal dilation of the athlete's pupils

- Fluid leaking from the athlete's ears
- Abnormal blood pressure
- Shock
- Loss of consciousness

Symptoms of spinal injury

- Back or neck pain
- Tingling or lack of feeling in the upper or lower limbs
- Muscle spasm in the neck and back
- Dizziness or confusion
- Headache

Management of spinal injuries

Due to the unknown severity of spinal injuries, all suspected cases should be treated as life threatening. The following key principles need to be considered by the sports trainer:

- DRSABCD
- Immobilisation of the athlete's neck and spine

All suspected spinal injuries require urgent emergency medical assessment.

IMMOBILISATION

If the athlete is lying in an awkward or unusual position on the ground, they should not be moved unless it is under the supervision of a medical professional such as a paramedic. If in an emergency the athlete does need to be moved, the following are the priorities for a sports trainer:

- airway, breathing and circulation
- minimising movement of the head and cervical spine
- minimising movement of the other spinal regions.

See Chapter 9 for more on spinal injuries.

Immobilisation of a suspected spinal injury should be attempted as soon as possible. A sports trainer should aim to maintain the head and neck in a neutral position and avoid unnecessary movement. This includes:

- applying an approved rigid cervical collar
- packing the head and neck of the athlete in sand or dirt
- using an improvised spinal collar such as towels if no better alternatives are available
- asking the athlete to remain calm and not move their head while you maintain gentle support by holding the head in a neutral position.

Brain and head injuries

The brain is a highly developed mass of nervous tissue that forms the upper end of the central nervous system. It has a soft and jelly-like structure and weighs about 1.4 kg in men and 1.25 kg in women, which is approximately 2% of total body weight. The human brain floats in cerebrospinal fluid within the rigid casing formed by the bones of the skull.

The brain is protected by:
- the skull
- a complex layer of connective tissue coverings between the brain and the skull
- a layer of fluid between these connective tissue coverings and the skull.

There are blood vessels (arteries and veins) within the brain as well as between the surface of the brain and the inner layer of the skull.

Nerve fibres passing to and from the brain join together at the base of the brain. The nerve tissue forms the spinal cord and exits the skull through a large hole in the base called the foramen magnum. The spinal cord lies within the spinal canal and is protected by the bony surrounds of the vertebral column.

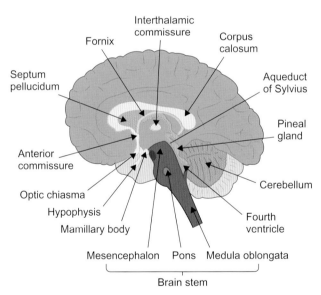

Figure 7.16 The brain

Brain injury in sport

Causes of sporting-related brain injury include a blow to the head or face or the head either coming to a sudden stop or being propelled forwards suddenly (acceleration/deceleration injuries).

All suspected brain injuries must be treated with the utmost seriousness and in strict accordance with established medical procedures, such as those adopted by sports such as the International Rugby Board (IRB), the Fédération Internationale de Football Association (FIFA) and the Australian Football League (AFL).

CONCUSSION

Concussion can be common in collision and contact sports. Concussion is a complex pathophysiological process affecting the brain that is caused by traumatic biomechanical forces. It is sometimes, but not always, associated with a loss or reduced level of consciousness.

For any suspected concussion, sports trainers are strongly advised to become familiar with and follow the protocols described in SCAT 2, the Sideline Concussion and Assessment Tool (see below).

CONTUSION AND COMPRESSION

Bleeding inside the skull can cause swelling and place pressure on the brain, leading to a loss of consciousness, coma or death. Milder forms of brain tissue contusion can cause symptoms similar to those of concussion but that tend to last longer.

DIRECT TRAUMA

This involves damage directly to the brain tissue from an associated closed or penetrating skull fracture, usually as the result of a direct trauma from an object or implement.

Signs of brain injury
- Loss of consciousness or reduced consciousness
- Poor coordination
- Loss of balance
- Dilated pupils
- Fluid leaking from the ears
- Vomiting
- Convulsions or seizure
- Slurred speech
- Amnesia or poor concentration

Symptoms of brain injury
- Headache – often low grade and persistent
- Dizziness/vertigo
- Nausea
- Tinnitus (ringing in the ears)
- Confusion/amnesia
- Irritability
- Fogginess/slowness/light-headedness
- Blurred or double vision
- Disorientation

Management of brain injury
If any of the above signs or symptoms are present:
- Send for medical assistance immediately.
- Initiate DRSABCD.
- Appropriately immobilise the athlete.

All suspected head injuries require removal from the field of play. Following any suspected or actual brain injury, medical clearance from a doctor must be obtained before allowing an athlete to return to competition or training.

Assessing brain injuries in athletes

The SCAT 2 Sideline Concussion and Assessment Tool is a pocket-sized card summary listing signs and symptoms of concussion, including those listed above, as well as memory and balance assessment tools that can indicate the presence of a brain injury.

To test **memory function** SCAT 2 recommends asking questions such as:

- What venue are we at today?
- Which half is it now?
- Who scored last in this game?
- What team did you play last week/game?
- Did your team win the last game?

Failing to answer all questions correctly may suggest a concussion.

Balance testing is also recommended using the tandem stance test. This test is described on the SCAT 2 card.

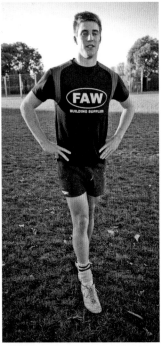

Figure 7.17 The tandem test for balance

Head injury form

A head injury form should be used by a sports trainer. The form contains important information that should be given to any athlete who has suffered a head injury. The athlete's parent/guardian should be advised to be watchful over the next 48 hours for any symptoms that indicate the need for urgent medical attention. If over the next 48 hours:

- the athlete's symptoms are getting worse
- the athlete develops a severe headache
- the athlete experiences visual disturbance
- the athlete experiences nausea or vomiting
- the athlete has a seizure
- the athlete feels weakness, or numbness of arms or legs

the parent/guardian should seek emergency medical advice immediately.

Dental injuries

Blood supply to the head is abundant so any injury to the face or mouth can cause profuse bleeding. When providing any care, wear gloves to reduce the risk of blood-borne infections.

Dental injuries can also occur in conjunction with injuries such as fractures of the jaw or cheekbone, and may sometimes involve concussion or unconsciousness. In the case of tooth loss, only a permanent (second) tooth should be replaced into the socket and only if the athlete is conscious.

Immediate care provided by the sports trainer at the scene can significantly reduce the risk of permanent tooth loss or damage. With dental injuries all tooth fragments must be recovered; otherwise, a chest X-ray may be required to exclude inhalation of a tooth or tooth fragments.

Tooth avulsion

A tooth avulsion is when a tooth is dislodged completely from its socket. An avulsed tooth should be replaced in the socket as soon as possible. Teeth that are reinserted into their socket within 20 minutes have the best chance of surviving.

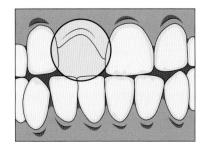

Tooth knocked out

Figure 7.18 Tooth avulsion

MANAGEMENT OF TOOTH AVULSION INJURIES

Locate the tooth and recover all tooth fragments. Holding the tooth by the crown (white part), carefully rinse dirt from the tooth with one of the following:

- best option – isotonic saline (in Dentist in a Box, available from SMA)
- second option – milk
- third option – water.

If you can reinsert the tooth, immediately replant the tooth in its socket using other teeth as a guide. Stabilise the replanted tooth if necessary by:
- best option – splinting disc (in Dentist in a Box, available from SMA)
- second option – biting into a clean piece of gauze or a clean handkerchief
- third option – holding the tooth in place by finger pressure.

The best option is to reinsert the tooth into its socket as this will keep it moist and in place. If this cannot be done for whatever reason, the next best options are listed as well below:
- best option – reinsert the tooth in its socket
- second option – place in a saline container (in Dentist in a Box)
- third option – place in a container of milk
- fourth option – place in the athlete's mouth.

For bleeding in the mouth, fold a small gauze square several times to make a pack that is placed over the wound. Instruct the athlete to close their teeth onto the pack, applying firm biting pressure to control bleeding, and consult a dentist as soon as possible.

Chipped or broken teeth

This is a very common injury that can affect any tooth. The injured tooth may be painful with temperature change or movement of air across the tooth surface when breathing through the mouth. Covering the exposed area of tooth provides relief; using a splinting disc will reduce thermal stimulation. Bleeding from the inside of the mouth and lips can occur due to the jagged or broken edges of affected teeth.

Recover and store the broken tooth fragments to aid the dentist. Ensure the athlete consults a dentist as soon as possible.

Tooth loosened or pushed out of position (luxation)

A permanent tooth may be loosened or moved slightly but not completely out of position. The management of tooth luxation includes:
- Move the tooth into the correct position as soon as possible.
- Stabilise the repositioned tooth if necessary by:
  - best option – using the splinting disc in Dentist in a Box
  - second option – biting into clean gauze or a clean handkerchief
  - third option – holding the tooth in place by finger pressure.
- Consult a dentist as soon as possible.

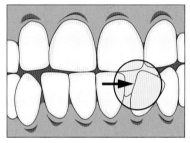
Tooth pushed out of position

Figure 7.20 Tooth luxation

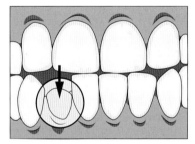
Tooth pushed into gum

Figure 7.21 Tooth intrusion

Tooth is pushed into the gum (intrusion)

Do not attempt to move the tooth; consult a dentist as soon as possible.

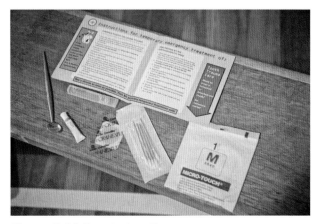

Figure 7.22 Dentist in a Box

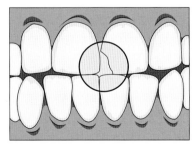
Chipped tooth

Figure 7.19 Chipped tooth

General rules relating to dental injuries

- Do not scrub the tooth.
- Do not touch the roots (yellow area); handle the tooth by the crown (white area) only.
- Do not scrape or rub the root surface.
- Do not let the tooth dry out.
- Do not store the tooth in dry gauze or tissue.
- Do not sterilise the tooth.
- Do not delay seeking treatment.

Chest and abdominal injuries

The trunk and the abdomen are usually injured in sport through contact with another body, implement, object or the environment. Contact and collision sports pose a greater potential for injury to these regions.

Chest injuries

When assessing an athlete with a chest injury, in addition to asking the general questions that the sports trainer would normally ask when performing TOTAPS, some other observations may provide indications that a chest injury or other cause of respiratory distress is present (see the table below). The athlete may also complain of pain when breathing, especially when taking a deep breath.

RESPIRATORY DISTRESS

Identifying respiratory distress	Adult Normal	Child Normal	Adult Abnormal	Child Abnormal
Normal respiratory rate	12–16 breaths per minute	20 breaths per minute	<10 breaths per minute *or* >20 breaths per minute	<15 breaths per minute *or* >25 breaths per minute
Respiratory rhythm (observe athlete's chest)	Rise and fall of chest is regular and even	Rise and fall of chest is regular and even	Rise and fall of chest is irregular and uneven	Rise and fall of chest is irregular and uneven
Respiratory effort (observe athlete's chest and neck)	During quiet respiration, there is usually only a small amount of chest movement	During quiet respiration, there is usually only a small amount of chest movement	▪ Marked chest movement ▪ Use of other accessory muscles to help get air in and out of the lungs (in the neck, abdomen and ribs)	▪ Marked chest movement ▪ Use of other accessory muscles to help get air in and out of the lungs (in the neck, abdomen and ribs)
Appearance	Calm and quiet	Calm and quiet	Breathing will be anxious and distressed May appear to be fighting for air or completely exhausted	Breathing will be anxious and distressed May appear to be fighting for air or completely exhausted
Ability to speak	Normally an athlete should speak in clear flowing sentences	Normally an athlete should speak in clear flowing sentences	Will be able to speak only in short sentences or single words	Will be able to speak only in short sentences or single words
Noises	Generally, no respiratory noises are audible	Generally, no respiratory noises are audible	Athletes may experience a cough, stridor, inspiratory/ expiratory wheeze or wet gurgling noises. In severe episodes the athlete may make no noise	Athletes may experience a cough, stridor, inspiratory/ expiratory wheeze or wet gurgling noises. In severe episodes the athlete may make no noise

Note: *An athlete may already have an elevated respiratory rate due to the exercise in which they have been participating. This can complicate observations, although the rate should return to normal within a few minutes after physical activity has ceased.*

COMMON SPORT-RELATED CHEST INJURIES

If there is local bony tenderness in the chest, manage the athlete as if there is a fractured rib, especially if taking a deep breath aggravates the pain. Very occasionally, an athlete who sustains a fractured rib may also be at risk of the fractured rib penetrating a lung, which could cause the lung to collapse. Initially, there may be few signs and symptoms of the collapsed lung, other than that of the chest injury, although shortness of breath can occur either immediately or sometime after the injury. If there is shortness of breath that does not quickly resolve, call for emergency medical aid. Continue to reassure the athlete and encourage them to continue to breathe as normally as possible until advanced aid arrives.

Abdominal injuries

Although the incidence of significant injury to the internal abdominal organs is relatively low, such injuries can occur and can be life threatening if not recognised and treated quickly.

INTERNAL ABDOMINAL BLEEDING

With internal organ injuries, be aware of the following:

- The signs and symptoms may develop over several hours and not be noticeable immediately.
- If any signs or symptoms of internal bleeding develop, the athlete must be urgently referred to emergency medical care or to a hospital.

Signs of internal abdominal bleeding

- Pale, cold and sweaty skin
- Increased heart rate
- Increased respiratory rate
- Abdominal swelling
- Loss of consciousness

Symptoms of internal abdominal bleeding

- Increasing abdominal pain
- Abdominal tenderness
- Nausea
- Possible thirst

Management of internal abdominal bleeding

- Send for urgent medical assistance and transfer the athlete to hospital.
- Rest the athlete quietly with the knees raised and resting at about 45° on pillows, bags or other soft objects.

- Do not give anything to eat or drink.
- Place a sheet, blanket or space blanket over the athlete to keep them warm.

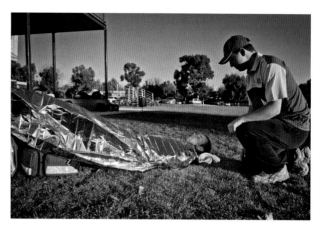

Figure 7.23 Managing suspected internal abdominal bleeding

Winding

Athletes who have been winded from a knock to the chest or abdomen may require treatment, although this is rarely an emergency. Winding typically occurs after a blow to the stomach or the back around the solar plexus, which is a cluster of nerves behind the stomach that influences respiration. Winding can also occur with any impact that temporarily interferes with or interrupts normal respiration.

Signs of winding

- Difficulty breathing
- Inability to speak
- Vomiting

Symptoms of winding

- Nausea

Management of winding

- Reassure the athlete.
- Help the athlete into a comfortable position.
- Encourage the athlete to take slow, deep breaths.
- Remain with the athlete until the breathing difficulty resolves.
- If the breathing difficulty does not improve in a few minutes, seek medical attention.
- Lay the unconscious athlete on their side in the lateral position, ensuring the airway remains clear, and continue to monitor the athlete's breathing.

When an athlete is winded, there is also potential for a rib fracture, lung damage or internal organ damage. This can be indicated by the signs listed in the relevant sections above.

The sports trainer should keep this in mind while observing the athlete over the next few hours. If any such signs occur, the athlete should not play contact sport until a doctor has assessed and cleared them to play.

Injuries to male external genitalia (testes and scrotum)

The testes are very soft tissue and are liable to damage. The testes are contained in a very tough fibrous coat lying within the skin of the scrotum to protect them as they lie outside the abdominal wall. A blow to the testes, which may occur in a variety of sports, is at first very painful and can cause the following signs and symptoms in an athlete.

Signs of injury to male genitalia

- Nausea
- Slow pulse
- Fainting or near fainting

Symptoms of injury to male genitalia

- Testicular pain
- Central abdominal pain

Usually these symptoms slowly settle and there is no cause for concern. However, as this is a soft tissue injury, the affected tissue may swell. Swelling may cause further compression of testicular tissue and increase pain. In some cases more serious injury can also occur, including rotation of the testes within the scrotum.

Management of injury to genitalia

- Rest the athlete with some discretion if in public view.
- **RICER** and **NO HARM** – please note that ice should be used carefully in this situation, as it may be more painful than the actual injury. Instead, advise the athlete to cool the area using a cold compress or a wet towel.

If the pain does not settle or if it increases over the next hour or so, the athlete should be referred for medical assessment. If the pressure continues to increase, there is a threat to the ongoing viability of the testes and an operation may be required, although this is unusual. If an operation is required, it usually needs to be performed within 4 hours of the incident if testicular function is to be preserved.

Environmental influences on sporting injuries

Athletes are commonly affected by illnesses arising from heat or cold. If not managed promptly and appropriately, these illnesses can become serious.

During exercise, the body produces a lot of heat. This heat must be lost or serious problems can occur. When exercising, it is important that the body's core temperature (internal temperature) is maintained within a narrow range. When the core temperature moves outside of this range, the body's capacity to perform activity will be reduced. When exercising in warm conditions temperature control becomes more difficult. In cooler climates, heat loss is not usually a problem but, if it is very cold, the body may not produce enough heat to keep the core temperature within an acceptable range.

How the body loses and gains heat

The body can lose or gain heat in several ways.

EVAPORATION

The major means by which the body loses heat during exercise is by evaporation of sweat from the skin. Evaporation is the process of converting liquid to gas. On hot and humid days, it is more difficult to cool the body by evaporation because the air is already saturated with water, which reduces the capacity for evaporation.

RADIATION

Heat can radiate from a warm object to a cooler one. In a cold climate, athletes will radiate heat to the environment surrounding them. During exercise on a warm day an athlete will gain heat from the surrounding environment.

CONVECTION

Airflow across the body results in heat loss by convection. Cold, windy conditions increase heat loss by convection. Athletes should be aware of the increased potential for heat loss by this method when exercising in these conditions. Clothing also influences heat transfer by convection.

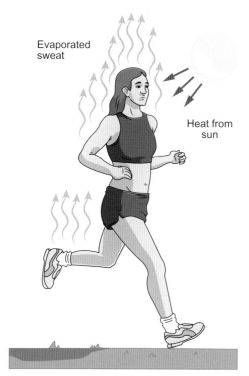

Figure 7.24 Evaporation

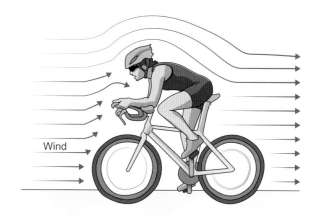

Figure 7.25 Convection

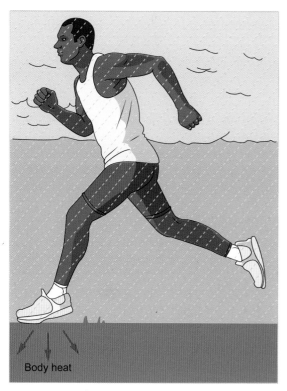

Figure 7.26 Radiation

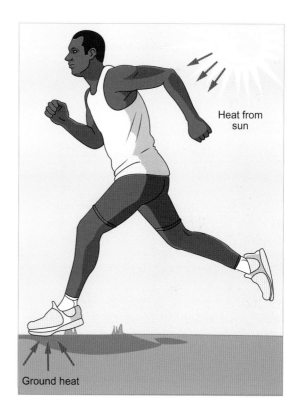

CONDUCTION

Heat is transferred when two objects at different temperatures contact each other; for example, an athlete will lose heat to the environment on a cold morning. Conduction is particularly important when exercising in water. Water is an effective conductor of heat; therefore, body heat will be lost very quickly in cool water.

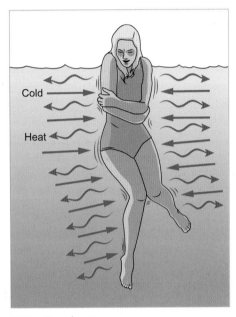

Figure 7.27 Conduction

Regulating body temperature

CHANGING THE AMOUNT OF BLOOD FLOW TO THE SKIN

If the body is cold, blood flow will decrease to the periphery (hands, feet and ears) and to the skin. If the core temperature is too hot, the body will dilate the blood vessels to increase the blood flow to the skin. Increased blood flow to the skin brings heat to the body surface where it will be lost, allowing cooling of deeper structures. Remember that the more blood is committed to transporting heat to the body surface, the less is available to the working muscles.

SWEATING

Most athletes sweat profusely to control their body temperature. Large quantities of water can be lost as sweat when exercising in the heat. This fluid must be replaced to allow the body to effectively control its temperature and function normally. If the fluid is not replaced, dehydration can occur, which will limit the body's ability to sweat and lose heat and will therefore diminish performance.

SHIVERING

If the temperature is cold, the body will attempt to produce heat by shivering. Shivering interferes with performance and should be avoided. Wearing appropriate clothing will help prevent this response.

Heat illness

High intensity exercise in a hot environment, with the associated elevation of body temperature, can lead to heat illness. Heat illness in sport can present as **heat cramps, heat exhaustion** or the more severe **heat stroke.**

The following sections on heat-related illness and its management are taken from the SMA Hot Weather Guidelines, which can be found on the website (www.sma.org.au).

Heat cramps

Heat cramps are associated with strenuous exercise or physical activity and can be extremely painful. They occur when too much salt has been lost through sweating and do not only occur in hot weather conditions. Athletes on salt-restricted diets and certain medications are especially susceptible to heat cramps.

Signs and symptoms of heat cramps include painful limb or stomach cramps, thirst, fatigue, dizziness, nausea and excessive sweating.

To manage heat cramps, have the athlete cease all physical activity and rest in a cool, shaded area. Give the athlete small amounts of water, fruit juice or sports drink. Seek medical advice if the cramps do not subside in approximately 1 hour.

Heat exhaustion

- Characterised by a high heart rate, dizziness, headache, loss of endurance/skill, confusion and nausea.
- The skin may still be cool/sweating, but there will be signs of developing vasoconstriction (e.g. pale colour).
- The rectal temperature may be up to 40°C and the athlete may collapse on stopping activity. Rectal temperature should only be measured by a doctor or nurse.

To avoid heat exhaustion, if people feel unwell during exercise they should immediately cease activity and rest. Further benefit comes if the rest is in a shaded area with some passing breeze (from a fan if necessary) and if the person takes extra hydration. Misting or spraying with water can also help.

Heat stroke

- Characteristics are similar to heat exhaustion but with a dry skin, confusion and collapse.
- Heat stroke may arise in an athlete who has not been identified as suffering from heat exhaustion and has persisted in further activity.

- Core temperature measured in the rectum is the only reliable method of diagnosing heat stroke in a collapsed athlete.

This is a potentially fatal condition and must be treated immediately. It should be assumed that any collapsed athlete is in danger of heat stroke.

The best first-aid measures are 'strip/soak/fan':

- Strip off any excess clothing.

- Soak with water.

- Fan.

- Ice placed in the groin and armpits is also helpful.

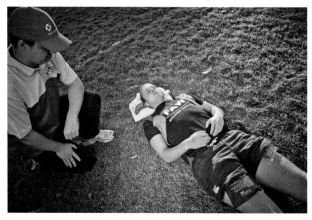

Figure 7.30 Ice packs near major arteries for heat stroke

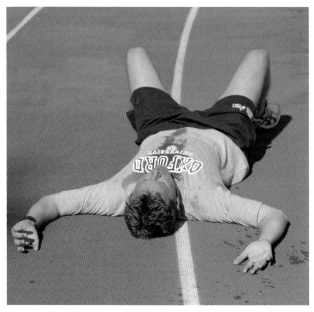

Figure 7.28 Signs of heat cramps

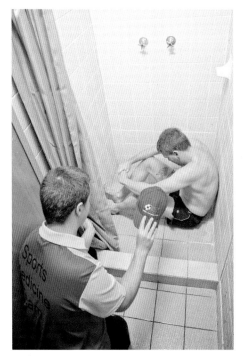

Figure 7.29 Initial management of heat exhaustion includes cold showers and fanning

The aim is to reduce body temperature as quickly as possible. The athlete should immediately be referred to a medical professional for treatment.

Important: heat exhaustion/stroke can still occur even in the presence of good hydration.

Dehydration

Dehydration is fluid loss that occurs during exercise, mainly due to perspiration and respiration. It makes an athlete more susceptible to fatigue and muscle cramps. Inadequate fluid replacement before, during and after exercise will lead to excessive dehydration and may lead to heat exhaustion and heat stroke. Even a small degree of dehydration will cause a decrease in performance. Remember to not only consider dehydration in players but also in umpires, officials and volunteers.

To avoid dehydration, SMA recommends that:

- Before exercise athletes should drink approximately 300–500 mL (2 glasses) every 30 minutes.

- During training/competition athletes should drink 250 mL every 15 minutes.

- After training athletes should continue to drink until the urine is clear.

Suitable drinks include cool water or sports drinks.

For more information, refer to SMA's DRINK UP brochure available on the website (http://www.smartplay.com.au).

Factors affecting heat illness

The tables in the following sections provide estimates of risks related to the weather and guidelines on managing activity in order to minimise heat stress.

ENVIRONMENTAL FACTORS

1 Temperature

Heat stress increases with increases in air temperature, but be aware that there are no clear demarcations in risk between temperature ranges. At relative humidity levels above those indicated in the tables, stress increases markedly.

Ambient temperature

This is the most easily understood guide available and is most useful on hot, dry days.

Ambient temperature	Relative humidity	Risk of heat illness	Possible management for sustained physical activity
15–20°C		Low	Heat illness can occur in distance running Caution over-motivation
21–25°C	Exceeds 70%	Low–moderate	Increase vigilance Caution over-motivation
26–30°C	Exceeds 60%	Moderate	Moderate early pre-season training Reduce intensity and duration of play/training Take more breaks
31–35°C	Exceeds 50%	High–very high	Uncomfortable for most people Limit intensity, take more breaks Limit duration to less than 60 minutes per session
36°C and above	Exceeds 30%	Extreme	Very stressful for most people Postpone to cooler conditions (or cooler part of the day) or cancellation

Wet Bulb Globe Temperature (WBGT) index

Further guidance might be gained from what is known as the Wet Bulb Globe Temperature (WBGT) index. The WBGT is useful when humidity is high. The Bureau of Meteorology (BOM) produces ambient and WBGT readings for many locations in Australia. You can check these readings and a guide for the relative risk for your location on the BOM website (www.bom.gov.au).

WBGT	Risk of thermal injury	Possible modifying action for vigorous sustained activity
<20°C	Low	Heat illness can occur in distance running Caution over-motivation
21–25°C	Moderate–high	Increase vigilance Caution over-motivation Moderate early pre-season training intensity and duration Take more breaks
26–29°C	High–very high	Limit intensity Limit duration to less than 60 minutes per session
30°C and above	Extreme	Consider postponement to a cooler part of the day or cancellation (allow swimming)

2 Duration and intensity of an event

- The combination of extreme environmental conditions and sustained vigorous exercise is particularly hazardous for an athlete. The greater the intensity of the exercise, the greater the risk of heat-related symptoms (e.g.

distance running is more of a problem than stop-start team events).

- The rotation of players and officials may be considered.
- Reducing playing time and extending rest periods, with opportunities to rehydrate during the event, would help to safeguard the health of participants.
- The provision of extra water for wetting the face, clothes and hair is important.
- A fan to enhance air movement would be beneficial.

3 Conduct of competition and training (hydration and interchange opportunities)

- Associations may consider dividing games into shorter playing periods, rather than halves, to allow for extra breaks.
- Coaches may consider alternative training times and venues during hot weather.
- Remember, even 5 minutes rest can cause a significant reduction in core temperatures.
- It is important to consider the welfare of officials as well as players.

4 Time of day

Avoid the hottest part of the day (usually 11 a.m.– 3 p.m.). Scheduling events outside this time should be a consideration for any summer competition, training or event, regardless of the temperature.

5 Local environment

- Radiant heat from surfaces such as black asphalt or concrete can exacerbate hot conditions.

- The type of exercise surface and the amount of sunlight vary significantly with different sporting activities and must be analysed for each individual sport.
- An air-conditioned indoor venue will provide less of a problem. A hot indoor venue or an outside venue without shade cannot be considered an acceptable environment.
- Airflow should be considered, including fans in change rooms or appropriately placed elsewhere.

Air movement decreases heat stress; however, a following wind can increase problems for runners or cyclists by actually reducing air movement.

HOST (PERSONAL) FACTORS

1 Clothing

The type of clothing is vital in minimising health risks associated with exercise in heat. Fabrics that minimise heat storage and enhance sweat evaporation should be selected. Lightweight, light-coloured and loose-fitting clothes made of natural fibres or composite fabrics with high wicking (absorption) properties that provide for adequate ventilation are recommended as the most appropriate clothing to wear in the heat. This clothing should complement the existing practices in Australia for protecting the skin against permanent damage from the sun. These recommendations apply to the clothing worn by players, umpires, other officials and volunteers.

Protective clothing

If clothing is worn for protective reasons, ensure that it is worn only while actually training and competing in hot weather. Some examples include leathers in motorcycling and mountain biking and protective equipment for hockey goalkeepers and softball and baseball umpires. Remove non-breathable clothing as soon as possible if the participants or officials are feeling unwell in hot conditions. Start cooling the body immediately via ventilation and/or a cool spray, such as a soaker hose or a hand-held spray, and a fan.

2 Acclimatisation of the participants

- Acclimatisation is necessary for umpires, other officials and volunteers as well as players.
- Preparation for exercise under hot conditions should include a period of acclimatisation to those conditions, especially if the athlete is travelling from a cool/temperate climate to compete in hot/humid conditions.
- It has been reported that children will acclimatise more slowly than adults.
- Regular exercise in hot conditions will facilitate adaptation, thus helping to prevent the athlete's performance deteriorating or the

athlete suffering from heat illness during later competitions. Sixty minutes acclimatisation activity each day for 7–10 days provides substantial preparation for safe exercise in the heat.

3 Fitness levels/athletic abilities of participants

- A number of physical/physiological characteristics of the athlete will influence the capacity to tolerate exercise in the heat, including body size and endurance fitness.
- In endurance events, accomplished but non-elite runners striving to maximise their performance may suffer from heat stress. The potential for heat-related illnesses is exacerbated if they have not acclimatised to the conditions and have failed to hydrate correctly.
- Overweight and unconditioned athletes, umpires, officials and volunteers will generally also be susceptible to heat stress.

4 Age and gender of participants

- Female participants may suffer more during exercise in the heat because of their greater percentage of body fat.
- Young children are especially at risk in the heat. Prior to puberty, their sweating mechanism, which is essential for effective cooling, is poorly developed. The ratio between weight and surface area in the child is also such that the body absorbs heat rapidly in hot conditions.
- In practical terms, child athletes must be protected from over-exertion in hot climates, especially with intense or endurance exercises.
- Although children can acclimatise to exercise in the heat, they take longer to do so than adults. Coaches should be aware of this and limit training for non-acclimatised children during exposure to hot environments. Children tend to have a more 'common sense' approach to heat illness than adults. They 'listen to their bodies' more and will usually slow down or stop playing if they feel distressed in the heat. On no account should children be forced to continue sport or exercise if they appear distressed or complain about feeling unwell.
- Veteran participants may also not cope as well with exercise in the heat. Reduced cardiac function is thought to be responsible for this effect.
- The sweating capabilities of wheelchair-bound and spinal-cord-injured athletes may be impaired and this places them at risk of heat illness.

5 Predisposing medical conditions

- It is important to know if athletes, umpires, officials or volunteers have a medical condition or are taking medication that may predispose them to heat illness.

- Examples of illnesses that will put participants or officials at a high risk of heat illness include asthma, diabetes, pregnancy, heart conditions and epilepsy. Those using some medications and having limiting medical conditions may need special allowances.

- Participants and officials who present with an illness such as a virus, flu or gastrointestinal infection, or who are feeling unwell, are at an extreme risk of heat illness if exercising in moderate to hot weather.

- Participants or officials affected by drugs or alcohol may be at an extreme risk of heat illness if exercising in moderate to hot weather.

- SMA's publication, *Pre-exercise Health Check Guidelines,* should be consulted if preexisting medical conditions are suspected or if the participant has no recent record of activity. The Guidelines can be downloaded from the website (www.sma.org.au).

6 Other factors to consider

- Preventive measures can be undertaken to minimise heat injuries. Examples include the provision of shade, hats, appropriate sunscreen, spray bottles and drinking water.

- It is important to have trained personnel available to manage heat injuries and designated recovery areas for patients.

- In situations where heat problems may be expected, an experienced medical practitioner should be present.

Heat stroke is potentially life threatening. Any indication of this condition should be immediately referred for medical assessment.

Cold illness

Cold weather conditions also affect performance. Cold conditions can create health problems ranging from reduced performance due to over-cooling of exercising muscles to **hypothermia** and **frostbite**.

Hypothermia

Hypothermia is a condition in which the body loses more heat than it can generate, resulting in a fall in core temperature below 35°C. The effects of hypothermia include decreased cardiovascular performance that can initially cause a reduction in blood flow to the exercising muscles, which can negatively affect muscle performance. This can progress to more severe effects including insufficient circulation to maintain normal heart function, leading to collapse and possibly death.

Frostbite

Frostbite occurs when skin tissue freezes after exposure to cold weather. This condition happens when the body is exposed to temperatures below the freezing point of the skin. The nose, cheeks, ears, fingers and toes are most commonly affected. Many people with frostbite may also be experiencing hypothermia, so saving their lives is more important than preserving a finger or foot.

SYMPTOMS OF FROSTBITE

- Pain
- Burning
- Numbness
- Tingling
- Itching
- Cold sensations in the affected areas
- Loss of feeling in the affected areas

SIGNS OF FROSTBITE

- Cold, white and hard skin
- Mottled skin
- Swelling and blistering
- Skin that becomes red and blotchy when warmed
- Blood-filled blisters (severe frostbite)
- Regions of skin that appear white and frozen but, if you press on them, retain some resistance

With deep frostbite, there is an initial decrease in sensation that is eventually completely lost. Swelling and blood-filled blisters appear over white or yellowish skin that looks waxy and turns a purplish blue as it rewarms. The area is hard, has no resistance when pressed and may even appear blackened and dead.

FIRST AID FOR FROSTBITE

- DRSABCD.
- Seek shelter and reduce further exposure to the cold and wind.
- Keep the affected body part elevated in order to reduce swelling.
- Give the person warm, non-alcoholic, non-caffeinated fluids to drink.
- Apply a dry, sterile bandage, place cotton between any involved fingers or toes (to prevent rubbing) and take the person to a medical facility as soon as possible.
- Remove any wet or restrictive clothing and replace with dry clothing wherever possible.

- Wrap the person in blankets and warm the person's entire body.
- Do not rub the affected area.
- Do not expose the person to direct radiant heat such as a fire.
- Take the pressure off the affected area to prevent further damage; for example, do not allow the person to walk on frostbitten feet.
- Do not allow the person to smoke cigarettes, since nicotine constricts the blood vessels.
- Do not attempt to thaw the affected part if there is a chance of it being refrozen.
- Do not break blisters.
- Above all, keep in mind that the final amount of tissue destruction is proportional to the time it remains frozen, not to the absolute temperature to which it was exposed. Therefore, rapid transport to a hospital is very important.

THAWING THE AFFECTED AREA

Most frostbite damage occurs during or after rewarming or thawing of the affected tissues. Damage can occur when an area is rewarmed and exposed again to cold. Thawing is painful and should only be attempted when medical assistance is available. Thawing and refreezing is dangerous.

Factors affecting cold illness

There are several factors that can affect an athlete's performance and health in a cold climate; these are set out below.

WEATHER CONDITIONS

Obviously, cold climates and low air temperature will be a major contributing factor to cold illness. Strong winds in cool climates increase heat loss by convection, also known as the 'wind chill factor'. Windproof clothing is necessary in these conditions to reduce heat loss.

Heat loss by convection can also occur in athletes travelling at high speeds in cold conditions, such as skiers or cyclists. These athletes must protect themselves from convection heat loss by wearing appropriate clothing.

CLOTHING

To prevent cold-related illness:
- Wear clothing that is appropriate for the conditions (i.e., clothing that prevents heat loss and insulates the body).
- Dress in layers to trap heat and prevent heat loss.
- Add or remove layers according to the exercise level and conditions.

- Hoods allow heat loss from the head to be reduced and can be removed according to the exercise level and conditions.
- Have warm, dry clothing available to reduce cooling during breaks and after the game.
- Clothing should be made of a material that will insulate, such as wool.
- Wear waterproof clothing if it is raining or snowing.
- The head, face and neck should be covered to reduce heat loss.

AGE, PHYSICAL CONDITION AND PERIOD OF EXPOSURE

- The young and elderly are most susceptible to cold illness as their bodies are less adaptable to variations in temperature.
- People with a high level of fitness and physical conditioning are more resilient to cold illness.
- The period of exposure also plays a vital factor in cold-related illness as risk increases with the amount of time exposed to a cold environment.

Wound management in sport

Blood rules

Injuries to the skin are common in sport. Any break in the skin can be a source of infection of the injured player regardless of whether there is bleeding or not. Skin wounds can also potentially expose other players to blood borne infections from the injured player, although the risk of this occurring is low. To minimise the risk to both the injured player and others around them, all wounds should be treated as potentially infectious.

Most sports now have blood rules in place that usually include:
- If a player who is bleeding has blood on their clothing, they must immediately leave the playing field or court and seek medical attention.
- The bleeding must be stopped, the wound dressed and blood on the player's body must be cleaned off before they return to the game.
- Play must cease until all blood on the ground or equipment is cleaned up.

Types of wounds

Injuries to the skin and subcutaneous tissues vary in type and severity. Some of the types of wounds encountered in sport include the following:
- Abrasions – loss of the superficial layer of skin
- Lacerations – a deep, jagged edged cut

- Incisions – a deep cut with smooth edges caused by a sharp object
- Puncture wounds – a deep, penetrating injury that can carry foreign material below the skin
- Skin avulsion – tearing of the skin, usually causing significant loss of blood

Treatment of wounds in sport

When treating any wound sports trainers should treat all blood as potentially infectious and therefore try to avoid any contact with blood. They should always wear latex or plastic gloves.

For wounds where there is profuse bleeding, the first priority is to stop blood loss using the techniques described in the earlier section on serious bleeding. Once bleeding has stopped, clean around the wound site with saline or warm, soapy water, wiping away from the wound and gently removing any loose foreign bodies that may be present. Use fresh swabs to clean the wound area itself. Sterile saline can also be used to wash out wounds.

With correct immediate treatment and dressings appropriate to the type of wound, most wounds heal more quickly and with a lower risk of infection or other complications. For many types of wounds, covering them with an occlusive dressing that keeps the wound moist but protected from the outside environment has been found to be effective in improving healing time and quality of skin repair. Occlusive dressings can be combined with antibiotic creams to further reduce the risk of infection.

There are many approaches to the treatment of wounds; they vary according to the type of wound and the other specific factors that may be present. There is also a wide and ever-expanding range of products that can be used to treat wounds, each of which has a particular purpose or indication for use. Due to the frequency and variety of wounds in sport and the range of treatment options available, sports trainers are advised to seek further training in this field.

Chapter Eight

COMMON MEDICAL CONDITIONS AFFECTING ATHLETES

LEARNING OUTCOMES

Describe and manage a range of medical conditions affecting athletes.

1   Describe management techniques of athletes with known medical conditions.
2   Identify signs and symptoms of a range of viral medical conditions.
3   Identify signs and symptoms of a range of chronic medical conditions.

ASSESSMENT OF OUTCOMES

Underpinning knowledge

You may be asked a number of written or oral questions related to the management of medical conditions that may be exhibited by an athlete. You may also be asked to complete an online task or workbook with related activities.

Practical demonstration

You will be asked to demonstrate effective management strategies of a variety of medical conditions in a sporting context.

Scenario

You may be asked to identify a number of medical conditions and how you would manage them in a crisis situation. This may include prioritising conditions as they present.

Introduction

Some medical conditions are common in the general population and, therefore, can also be present in sports participants. Medical conditions can affect an athlete's performance. Similarly, performance can affect a medical condition. The sports trainer requires a basic understanding of common illnesses and medical conditions and how they can affect or be influenced by athletic performance.

Common medical conditions

The sports trainer is expected to have a sound knowledge of the following common medical conditions and their effects on sports participation:

- asthma
- diabetes
- epilepsy
- cardiovascular conditions
- viral infections
- chronic illness and injury.

These conditions, when medically controlled and supervised, may not preclude an athlete from participating in physical activity, but modification of their exercise program may be necessary. After diagnosis by a medical practitioner, each athlete should have an individual management plan that covers prevention and treatment of their condition. The sports trainer has an important role in ensuring the athlete follows their plan and assisting them to do so.

Medical management plans should take into consideration:

- the nature and severity of the illness
- potential risks to the athlete and to other participants
- the athlete's goals.

For the protection of the athlete and to assist the sports trainer, every athlete should:

- undertake a pre-competition medical assessment (PCMA) with their doctor. The pre-exercise screening system developed by SMA in conjunction with Exercise Sports Science Australia and Fitness Australia could also be used
- for athletes with medical conditions, obtain clearance from a medical practitioner before beginning a new season
- complete an athlete medical profile form that outlines their medical history
- notify the sports trainer of any changes to their condition or medications, including recent illnesses not of a chronic nature such as a virus or other infection.

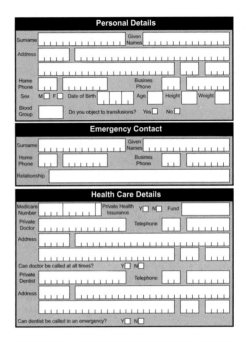

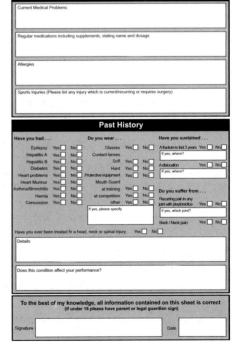

Figure 8.1 Athlete medical profile form (see Appendix C for a full-sized version)

Asthma

Asthma is the narrowing of the airways due to spasm and/or swelling of the airway walls, which restricts airflow and makes breathing difficult. There may also be an accumulation of mucus and fluid in the airways that contributes to the narrowing of the airways.

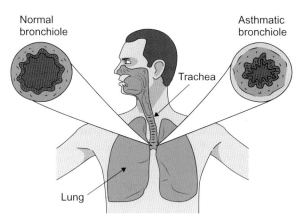

Figure 8.2 Normal airway versus asthma-affected airway

Some general triggers for asthma include:
- allergies, commonly including dust, pollens, grasses, lawn cuttings, animal hair
- cigarette smoke
- cold air
- certain medications, such as aspirin
- viral illnesses, including colds and flu
- altered emotional state, including stress.

Exercise-induced asthma (EIA) refers to asthma that is triggered during or shortly after exercise. EIA can vary from a mild cough to wheezing or to severe breathing difficulties. EIA may occur during exercise but is more likely to occur after exercise, usually up to 30 minutes after exercise.

During exercise, heat and water are lost from the airways and it is this cooling and dehydrating effect on the airways that is thought to trigger EIA. The more intense and the longer the duration of the exercise the more likely it is that EIA will occur.

Continuous activities such as distance running are more likely to induce EIA than stop/start activities such as soccer or netball. Cold and/or dry air can also affect people with asthma and the combination of this with exercise presents an added risk in sport.

It is important for all people with asthma to be prepared before exercising. This always involves an effective warm-up but may also include taking prescribed medication. Being physically and aerobically fit benefits all people, including people with asthma.

Signs of an asthma attack

There is often, but not always, a history of asthma. During an attack, the athlete may appear to have one or more of the following signs:
- difficulty breathing
- difficulty speaking
- shortness of breath
- noisy breathing, such as coughing or wheezing
- increased respiratory rate
- increased heart rate
- pale and sweaty skin
- quiet and slow responses
- in children, skin being sucked in around the base of the neck and between the ribs.

A severe attack can lead to:
- a blue tinge to the lips (cyanosis)
- unconsciousness.

Symptoms of an asthma attack

- Distress
- Anxiety
- Difficulty speaking
- Tiredness and exhaustion

In severe asthma attacks, the audible wheezing may subside as the condition worsens with very little air moving in and out of the lungs. This is an emergency. Never assume that a decrease in audible wheezing is a sign of improvement unless breathing also improves. If there are any signs of a severe attack, call an ambulance immediately and commence first aid following the usual DRSABCD principles.

Management of a severe asthma attack

- Sit the athlete comfortably upright. Be calm and reassuring.
- Help administer four puffs of a reliever or combination inhaler (Ventolin, Airomir, Epaq, Symbicort or Asmol).
- Relievers are best given through a spacer, if available. Use one puff at a time and ask the person to take four breaths from the spacer after each puff. Use the person's own inhaler if possible. If not, use the inhaler from the first aid kit or borrow one from someone else.
- Wait 4 minutes. If there is no improvement, give another four puffs, ensuring the person takes four breaths in and out through the spacer after each puff of medication.
- If there is little or no improvement, *call an ambulance immediately* and state that the athlete is having an asthma attack. Keep giving four puffs every 4 minutes until the ambulance arrives.

Note: *The protocol is the same for adults and children.*

If the athlete loses consciousness at any stage, place them on their side, make sure the airway is clear and monitor breathing and circulation. Start CPR if necessary.

RELIEVER MEDICATION WITH A SPACER

- Shake the inhaler and insert the mouthpiece into the spacer.
- Place the spacer mouthpiece in the person's mouth and fire one puff.
- Ask the person to breathe in and out normally for about four breaths.
- Repeat in quick succession until four puffs have been given.

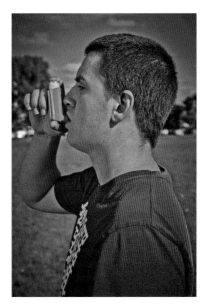

Figure 8.4 Reliever medication without a spacer is less effective

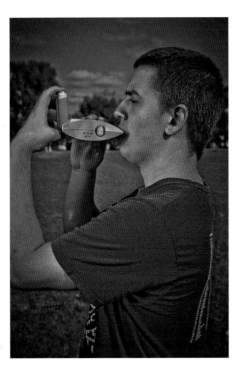

Figure 8.3 Reliever medication with a spacer

RELIEVER MEDICATION WITHOUT A SPACER

- Shake the inhaler.
- Place the puffer in the person's mouth. Fire one puff as the person inhales slowly and steadily.
- Ask the person to take four normal breaths.
- Repeat until four puffs have been given.

First asthma attack

- If someone collapses and appears to have difficulty breathing, *call an ambulance immediately*, whether or not the person is known to have asthma.
- Give four puffs of a reliever and repeat if there is no improvement.
- Keep giving four puffs every 4 minutes until the ambulance arrives.
- No harm is likely to result from giving a reliever to someone who does not have asthma.
- If a reliever is used for an athlete who is not known to have asthma, the athlete must be referred to a doctor for further assessment; this may confirm a diagnosis of asthma and thus require ongoing medical management.

Asthma medications

There are three types of medications prescribed for asthma:

1. reliever medications
2. preventive medications
3. combination medications.

RELIEVER MEDICATIONS

Reliever medications are taken 5–10 minutes prior to exercise and during exercise when necessary. They are available over the counter at most pharmacies. All sports trainers should carry at least one reliever inhaler and spacer in their sports medicine equipment. Reliever medications are blue/grey inhalers with the following product names: Ventolin, Airomir, Epaq and Asmol. Bricanyl, which is a dry powder reliever, is not recommended for first aid and can only be used by elite athletes if a Therapeutic Use Exemption (TUE) request has been submitted.

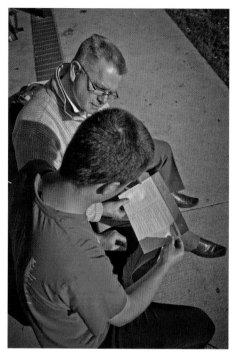

Figure 8.5 An asthma medication plan from a doctor is essential

PREVENTIVE MEDICATIONS

These are taken regularly and are prescription drugs that will not help when an athlete is having an asthma attack. They are:

- white with a blue cap (e.g. Intal)
- white with a red cap (e.g. Intal Forte)
- a brown turbuhaler (e.g. Pulmicort)
- burgundy (e.g. Qvar)
- orange (e.g. Flixotide)
- dark orange (e.g. Alvesco).

COMBINATION MEDICATIONS

These medications combine a preventer and a long-acting reliever in the same puffer. Combination medications are:

- red (e.g. Symbicort)
- purple (e.g. Seretide).

Asthma and the athlete

Well-controlled asthma should *not* prevent exercise and participation in most sports (however, people with asthma should not scuba dive). People with diagnosed asthma should have an *asthma management plan* or an *asthma action plan* that is established in conjunction with their doctor. The athlete, teammates, coach and the sports trainer should know this plan. The sports trainer should also encourage the person with asthma to:

- know the severity of their asthma
- exercise safely and regularly to improve fitness and lung function
- avoid trigger factors where possible
- perform at their best by using the right medication in the correct manner
- have their asthma checked regularly by their doctor – every 6 months
- have a ready supply of medication for use before, during and after exercise.

The sports trainer should identify the athletes in their team that have asthma and know their asthma management plan.

PRE-EXERCISE ADVICE

During pre-exercise, the athlete should avoid:

- allergy triggers, where possible (e.g. dust, pollens, grasses etc)
- exercising in cold air (e.g. early morning or late evening)
- vigorous exercise when the athlete has a viral infection
- any exercise if the athlete is wheezing or has a chest infection.

The athlete should always:

- warm up adequately to allow the body to adapt to changes in the weather; an indication of an adequate warm-up is a light sweat
- if advised by the doctor, take medication 5–10 minutes before exercise
- stretch after warming up.

Two different types of warm-up have been shown to be effective in reducing EIA:

- 5–7 sets of 30-second sprints with 30–60 seconds rest
- a brisk walk/slow jog for 20–30 minutes.

DURING EXERCISE ADVICE

- If asthma develops during exercise, stop the athlete and have them take their reliever medication.
- Do not allow the athlete to resume activity until all the signs and symptoms have subsided.

If the symptoms recur:

- use the reliever medication again
- do not allow the athlete to return to activity
- refer the athlete to their doctor
- do not encourage an athlete to 'run through' an asthma attack.

POST-EXERCISE ADVICE

Ensure an adequate cool-down takes place; i.e., 5–10 minutes of light activity followed by stretching.

If EIA continues, refer the athlete to their doctor, who may recommend:

- a change in medication
- regular preventive medication in the overall asthma management plan.

Further information

For more information on asthma, visit the National Asthma Council website at www.nationalasthma.org.au.

Diabetes

Diabetes is a disorder in which the body does not produce enough effective insulin to regulate blood sugar levels correctly. Insulin is a hormone that is needed to regulate the blood sugar levels in the body. In most instances, diabetes does not prevent a person from being able to participate in regular activity.

A regular exercise program will help to maintain blood sugar levels. A long-term regular exercise program may have considerable benefits to the diabetic, including decreased insulin dosages as well as increased wellbeing, flexibility, endurance and strength. The correct balance between diet, medication (oral or injection) and exercise can help control diabetes. The athlete should also be assessed regularly by their doctor.

If diabetic athletes overexert themselves or suddenly change their routine, their blood sugar levels may drop, which can lead to lead to serious consequences including shock or a diabetic coma.

Types of diabetes

There are two main types of diabetes:

1. Type 1 diabetes – it is believed that this is an autoimmune condition where the insulin cells in the pancreas fail. This condition typically presents before the age of 30 years and usually early in childhood. Type 1 diabetics require insulin replacement via injection, pen or pump to survive.

2. Type 2 diabetes – this is the most rapidly increasing medical condition in the world. It more often affects people over the age of 40 years and accounts for around 85% of all cases of diabetes. Lifestyle factors (lack of exercise and obesity) are the biggest contributing factors in developing type 2 diabetes. This condition may be controlled with diet, exercise and oral medication, but may require insulin-replacement therapy.

Another sub-type of diabetes is gestational diabetes, which occurs in 3–8% of pregnant women around the 24th to 28th week of pregnancy. This type of diabetes does not usually persist long after delivery. Most cases can be controlled by a good diet and exercise, but some women will require insulin.

People with diabetes are at risk of episodes of loss of consciousness due to:

- excessive lowering of the blood sugar level, known as hypoglycaemia; this occurs very quickly and needs urgent medical attention
- high blood sugar levels (hyperglycaemia); this usually occurs more slowly and is less likely to be seen by a sports trainer.

In any case of sudden, unexpected, unexplained loss of consciousness, there is a possibility that the person may have diabetes. Look for signs of injection marks on the lower abdomen or the front of the thighs. This is where most diabetics inject their insulin.

Signs of low blood sugar (hypoglycaemia)

- Pallor
- Excessive sweating
- Rapid pulse
- Seizures
- Altered state of consciousness or loss of consciousness

Symptoms of low blood sugar (hypoglycaemia)

- Feeling shaky or tremulous
- Anxiety
- Dizziness and loss of concentration
- Tingling around the lips
- Headache
- Confusion or disorientation, such that the diabetic is not able to help/treat themselves
- Hunger

Management of low blood sugar (hypoglycaemia)

- If the person is conscious, help them to eat some foods with fast-acting sugar, such as a sachet or lump of sugar, honey, fruit juice, glucose gel, sports drink, soft drink or jelly beans. Athletes with diabetes will usually carry suitable snacks with them.
- On recovery, make sure the person eats high-carbohydrate food (such as a sandwich, smoothie, yoghurt) and drinks some juice.
- On recovery, the athlete may need to be referred to their doctor to make sure that their diabetes is under good control.

If unconscious:

- call for emergency medical assistance immediately

- follow DRSABCD
- do not try to give the athlete anything by mouth.

Travelling with diabetic athletes

If an athlete with diabetes travels interstate or overseas, there are a number of considerations to take into account. If flying, medications, syringes, testing equipment and 80% of their insulin needs to be kept in their hand luggage and the remainder kept in their luggage in the aircraft hold. The excitement of a trip may affect an athlete's blood glucose levels so more frequent blood glucose testing is required.

Further information

For further information on diabetes, the Diabetes Australia website is www.diabetesaustralia.com.au/.

Epilepsy

Epilepsy is a condition in which various areas of the brain discharge spontaneously, resulting in a seizure. When a seizure (commonly referred to as a fit) occurs, the athlete may lose control of their body movements. Many conditions may cause individuals to have isolated seizures (e.g. head injury), although only recurrent seizures are diagnosed as epilepsy. The characteristic seizures in epilepsy are due to a disruption in normal brain functioning, with an abnormal discharge of activity causing disturbances in consciousness and/or movement.

There are two major types of seizures:

1 Grand mal seizures, which are sometimes described as the 'fits', are normally associated with shaking of the limbs and loss of consciousness. During the seizure, the person does not have control of their limbs and can cause damage to themselves or others. At this time, the person is unconscious and not breathing. These last for 3–5 minutes. The person is extremely tired afterwards.

2 Absence seizures, which only occur in children, disappear at about the age of 20. They are characterised by short (1- to 2-second) periods of absence (momentary losses of consciousness). These children may present with learning difficulties. Medications for these seizures work extremely well.

The sports trainer should know if any of their athletes have epilepsy. Information about their seizures, medications and any limitations recommended by their doctor should be obtained.

Epilepsy should not preclude an athlete from participating in sport, especially as modern medication has resulted in up to 80% of epileptics being seizure-free or only suffering infrequent episodes. For the remainder of people with epilepsy, the number of seizures can be considerably reduced; therefore, the sports trainer should encourage sporting participation at all levels from recreational to elite. However, some types of sport (archery, pistol shooting, scuba diving) may be less suitable for epileptics because of the potential danger to themselves or others.

Management of a seizure

- Remain calm and stay with the athlete.
- Do not restrain the athlete.
- Do not move the athlete unless they are in danger (e.g. from a roadway or if they are near fire or water). Athletes may be guided in their movements to a safer place or position. If seizures occur in wheelchairs or car seats, athletes should remain seated and protected from falling.
- Remove nearby objects that may cause injury to the athlete.
- Place something soft under the athlete's head.
- Time the duration of the seizure.
- After the seizure, place the athlete in the lateral position.
- Loosen any tight clothing the athlete is wearing.
- Do not put anything in the athlete's mouth.
- If the athlete vomits, put them in the lateral position immediately. Otherwise, do so upon recovery.
- Reassure the athlete until they have fully recovered.
- Call an ambulance if:
  - a seizure lasts longer than 5 minutes
  - a seizure is longer than usual for an individual
  - it is the athlete's first seizure
  - one seizure is followed quickly by another
  - the athlete is injured
  - the athlete has breathing difficulties after the seizure
  - the athlete is pregnant
  - the athlete has diabetes.
- Cover the athlete with a blanket or a sheet in case there is incontinence due to loss of bladder or bowel control.

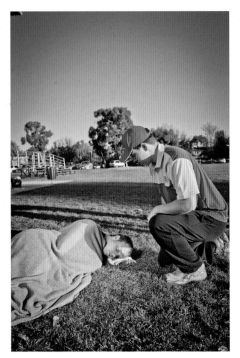

Figure 8.6 Athlete being monitored following a seizure

Seizures usually last from 1 to 3 minutes. Following these seizures, the athlete may be unconscious and must be monitored in the lateral position while waiting for transport to medical aid. The athlete may be very tired and wish to rest or sleep, have a headache and be confused or disoriented.

Considerations for athletes with epilepsy

- Fatigue – continuing to exercise when fatigued can induce a seizure. Encourage the athlete to monitor their program and stop before fatigue sets in.
- Cool-down – seizures are more likely to occur during cool-down than during the exercise program.
- Rapidly changing environments – flashing lights are likely to induce a seizure.
- Swimming or aquatic sports – these sports require close supervision and knowledge of how to handle a seizure in the water. A buddy system for swimmers is one way to increase the safety for epileptic athletes. If an athlete is having a seizure in water:
  - support them in the water with the head tilted so the face and head stay above the surface
  - remove them from the water as quickly as possible
  - check to see whether they are breathing; if not, begin CPR immediately
  - call an ambulance; even if the athlete appears to be fully recovered they should have a full medical examination

– inhaling water can cause lung or heart damage.

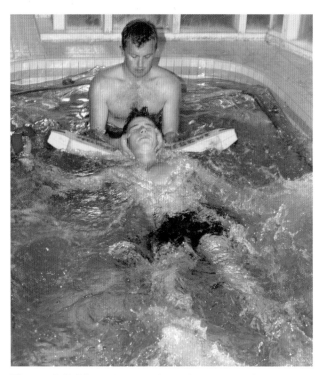

Figure 8.7 Managing a seizure in an aquatic environment

Cardiovascular emergencies

Cardiovascular emergencies in sport are fortunately extremely rare but require appropriate early recognition and management. The acute coronary syndromes sports trainers are most likely to see and be required to manage are cardiac chest pain and cardiac arrest. Sudden cardiac arrhythmia (SCA) is a rare condition in which life-threatening changes in heart function occur during sport in young athletes without a previously known risk or history of cardiac problems. Regardless of the cause of a disturbance to normal cardiac function, management by sports trainers should be the same: following the DRSABCD guidelines. Early notification to and response from emergency medical support will improve an athlete's management and ensure better outcomes for the athlete.

Players, coaches and sports trainers should be aware of sometimes subtle signs in athletes that could indicate cardiac risk factors. Symptoms can include chest pain or tightness, shortness of breath, irregular heartbeat, dizziness or fainting when exercising or tiring more quickly than similarly trained team mates. If any of these symptoms is present, ensure that the athlete consults their doctor for a proper medical evaluation before undertaking further training or competition. It is also important that athletes do not train hard or play when they are sick. Viral infections can increase the risk of cardiac events.

Certain lifestyle factors are known to be associated with narrowing of the coronary arteries and lead to higher risks of cardiovascular complications. Athletes with a higher risk of cardiovascular complications include those who:

- smoke
- have high blood pressure
- are obese
- have high blood cholesterol
- have an inactive lifestyle
- are male
- have certain diseases (e.g. diabetes).

Everyone should attempt to *prevent* the onset of coronary artery disease by eliminating the risk factors, where possible, from their lifestyle.

There are several cardiovascular emergencies that may present in athletes:

- angina
- hypertension
- heart attack
- stroke (cerebrovascular accident)
- acute exacerbation of chronic heart failure.

All of these conditions require immediate medical assistance. The sports trainer should commence appropriate first aid until more qualified personnel arrive.

Assessing perfusion status

The perfusion status assessment is made up of four observations that, when taken in the context of athletes presenting with a problem, help determine whether the cardiovascular system is functioning adequately. The four observations are of the pulse, conscious state, skin and temperature. Any athlete who has changes to two or more of the four categories should be considered less than adequately perfused. Such a person is considered to be 'actual time-critical' and in urgent need of medical attention to survive.

PULSE

Using the pads of two or three fingers (but not the thumb), palpate either the carotid or radial artery. Count the pulse for 15 seconds then multiply by 4 to obtain the athlete's pulse rate per minute. The normal *resting* pulse rate for an adult is 60–100 beats per minute. A faster or slower rate than this may indicate the heart is not pumping as efficiently as normal or that there is not enough oxygen being supplied to the tissues.

CONSCIOUS STATE

Under normal circumstances, an athlete should be alert and orientated in time and place. An altered level of consciousness may indicate a lack of oxygen

delivered to the brain, which may occur if the heart is not pumping effectively. The Glasgow Coma Scale can be used to assess an athlete's conscious state.

		Score
Eye opening		
Spontaneous	O	4
To speech	O	3
To pain	O	2
None	O	1
Best verbal response		
Oriented conversation	O	5
Confused conversation	O	4
Inappropriate words	O	3
Inappropriate sounds	O	2
None	O	1
Best motor response		
Obeys commands	O	6
Localises pain	O	5
Withdrawal from pain	O	4
Abnormal flexion	O	3
Abnormal extension	O	2
None	O	1

Figure 8.8 Glasgow Coma Scale

SKIN AND TEMPERATURE

Observe the athlete's skin colour and feel it for warmth. An adult's skin is normally warm (depending on environmental factors), pink and dry. If the athlete's skin is pale or cyanosed (blue looking) or cool and clammy (excluding environmental factors), it may indicate that the body is compensating for something and supplying only the vital organs with oxygen. Pale, cool, clammy skin is indicative of a reduced blood supply to the skin.

Diving emergencies

There are two main types of diving emergencies:

1. Air embolism (arterial gas embolism) – the more immediate condition that a sports trainer may need to treat is caused by a too rapid and uncontrolled ascent. Symptoms usually occur within 5 minutes of surfacing. In severe cases, symptoms will occur within 30 seconds of surfacing, causing unconsciousness with a high probability of drowning.

2. Decompression illness – usually presents after a dive and it is less likely that a sports trainer will need to treat this illness. Symptoms, which can often be very mild, can develop up to 48 hours after a dive, especially if air travel is undertaken within this timeframe.

Signs of an air embolism

- Irregular breathing or absence of breathing
- Altered level of consciousness
- Bloody froth from the mouth or nose
- Collapse
- Shock

Symptoms of an air embolism

- Cough
- Chest pain
- Weakness or paralysis
- Blurred or disturbed vision
- Dizziness and disorientation

Signs of decompression illness

- Paralysis or muscle weakness
- Rash
- Difficulty breathing
- Loss of balance
- Loss of consciousness
- Shock

Symptoms of decompression illness

- Fatigue
- Headache
- Malaise
- Itchy skin
- Joint pain
- Abdominal pain
- Disorientation
- Dizziness/vertigo
- Altered speech or higher brain function
- Numbness or tingling

Management of diving emergencies

- Immediately place the diver flat on their back with the head level with the heart. Do not elevate the head.
- Follow DRSABCD.
- Resuscitate the diver, if necessary.
- If trained personnel are present, administer oxygen in the highest concentration possible:
  - Use an anaesthetic mask with airbag and an oxygen reservoir bag, if available.
  - Deliver oxygen direct to the diver's demand valve, if a connection is available.
- Reassure the diver.
- Remain with the diver and send others for help (dial 000 for immediate assistance and then contact the Divers Emergency Service on 1800 088 200 to speak to a doctor experienced in diving emergencies).

Before diving

Everyone intending to take up diving should first have a medical examination from a doctor experienced in diving medicine.

Note: A list of these medical professionals is available at www.spums.org.au.

Viral infections

Viral infections are the most common infections affecting both the general community and sports people. The symptoms and effects viruses have on people vary in severity, ranging from minor sniffles to a sore throat to severely debilitating illness such as chronic fatigue syndrome and even death in the case of hepatitis and AIDS.

Simple upper respiratory tract viral infections (cold and flu)

The following are the common signs and symptoms of simple upper respiratory tract viral infections that the sports trainer will see and hear.

SIGNS OF SIMPLE UPPER RESPIRATORY TRACT VIRAL INFECTIONS

- Fever (which may go up and down over hours)
- Flushed or pale skin
- A generally unwell appearance

SYMPTOMS OF SIMPLE UPPER RESPIRATORY TRACT VIRAL INFECTIONS

- Fatigue
- Sore throat
- Running nose
- Cough
- Mild shortness of breath
- Headache
- Hot and cold sweats (rigors)

Simple gastrointestinal tract viral infections

The following are the common symptoms and signs of simple gastrointestinal tract viral infections that the sports trainer will observe.

SYMPTOMS OF SIMPLE GASTROINTESTINAL TRACT VIRAL INFECTIONS

- Feeling unwell
- Nausea
- Abdominal pain
- Feeling bloated

SIGNS OF SIMPLE GASTROINTESTINAL TRACT VIRAL INFECTIONS

The signs of simple gastrointestinal tract viral infections are often hard to find even in severe cases.

- Abdominal tenderness; a doctor would need to differentiate viral gastroenteritis (inflamed stomach and intestines) from early surgical problems such as appendicitis and gall bladder disease.
- The athlete is often very pale and may develop sunken eyes (a late characteristic of dehydration that requires urgent emergency medical assistance).
- Vomiting or diarrhoea.

Viral illness and its effect on an athlete

MILD VIRAL ILLNESS (SIGNS AND SYMPTOMS BUT NO FEVER)

There is little risk of complication if a doctor's diagnosis is that:

- the viral illness is mild
- the athlete feels they are able to play
- an adequate period of rest is available afterwards (i.e., the athlete is playing in a weekly competition)
- the event is not exhausting.

Current research suggests that playing sport while suffering from a mild viral illness may prolong the illness for 1–2 days longer than if the athlete had rested, although this is difficult to prove.

MODERATE VIRAL ILLNESS (SIGNS AND SYMPTOMS AND MILD FEVER)

Exercise performed during viral illness requires greater cardiopulmonary effort, which will have a detrimental effect on performance. If the viral illness is moderate, the athlete will usually not perform well. Playing sport with a moderate viral illness will almost certainly prolong the course of the illness.

SEVERE VIRAL ILLNESS (SIGNS AND SYMPTOMS AND INCREASED FEVER)

If the viral illness is severe, there is a definite risk of prolonging the condition as well as suffering complications such as:

- pericarditis, an inflammation of the lining of the heart
- abnormal heart rhythm, which is a risk factor for sudden death.

EXERCISE AND VIRAL ILLNESS

Australian researchers are currently amongst the world leaders in research into this area. It appears that:

- Mild exercise helps to stimulate the body's defence mechanism (immune system):
  - in fighting off viral infections such as colds
  - in helping the body recover from viral infections.
- Intense exercise appears to temporarily inhibit some aspects of the immune system, so there may be a period of increased susceptibility to viral illness associated with heavy training.
- Elite athletes who are consistently in heavy training seem to be a little more vulnerable to infection when training loads are reduced (e.g. when tapering before a competition and when psychological stress is increased due to the impending competition).
- Stress of competition, as well as the physical aspects of the sport, can impair immune functioning.

MANAGEMENT OF VIRAL ILLNESS

- Have the athlete cease all physical activity.
- Have the athlete seek medical advice regarding their condition.
- Do not permit the athlete to return to training or competition without a medical clearance.

Specific viral illnesses

Hepatitis A

Hepatitis A is probably the most common type of hepatitis in young people. It is caused by infection with the hepatitis A virus (Hep A), which is transmitted by the faecal–oral route.

SIGNS OF HEPATITIS A

- Signs of a viral illness
- Vomiting
- Yellowing of the skin (jaundice), which appears one week after the viral illness signs

SYMPTOMS OF HEPATITIS A

- Fever
- Abdominal pain
- Loss of appetite
- Nausea

MANAGEMENT OF HEPATITIS A

Any athlete who presents with these symptoms should be referred to a doctor for diagnosis and appropriate management, which usually involves:

- rest until the symptoms subside
- gradual resumption of activity, as tolerated.

Full recovery is expected. Hepatitis A vaccinations are available that help to reduce the severity of the illness.

PREVENTION OF HEPATITIS A

Anyone in close contact with those suffering Hep A may be given the Hep A vaccine as a preventive measure.

If an athlete is confirmed as suffering from Hep A, serious consideration should be given to immunising the other team members.

Hepatitis B

Hepatitis B (Hep B) has potentially serious long-term complications. It is transmitted sexually (by mixing of body fluids) or by direct contact with contaminated needles or infected blood. Note that hepatitis B can be transmitted by blood that has already dried.

Exercise should be avoided until symptoms have completely disappeared and blood tests return to normal. Occasionally, athletes with Hep B develop potentially life-threatening liver problems.

Those infected with the Hep B virus may remain 'carriers' for life. Exposure to the Hep B virus is a potential problem in contact sport. Sports Medicine Australia has published infectious diseases guidelines for the reduction of the risk of transmitting infectious diseases. Preventive immunisation with Hep B vaccine should be compulsory for all athletes and sports trainers in contact sports that have a high incidence of blood-exposed injuries. The National Health and Medical Research Council (NHMRC) guidelines for immunisation include recommendations for all Australians to be immunised against hepatitis B.

Hepatitis C

Hepatitis C (Hep C) is the major causative agent of post-transfusion hepatitis. The transmission and recognition resembles that of Hep B. The major method of transmission is through sexual contact or blood products.

The chance of being infected by a Hep C carrier is low, but if infection occurs there is a high rate of chronic complications. There is no vaccine available for Hep C.

Human immunodeficiency virus (HIV)

Human immunodeficiency virus (HIV) is a potentially lethal virus transmitted sexually or by contact with blood or blood products. Following infection with HIV, a flu-like illness often develops. This is followed by an asymptomatic period that may last months or years. Acquired immunodeficiency syndrome (AIDS) subsequently develops; this presents in a variety of ways associated with suppression of immunity, including AIDS-associated diseases such as severe pneumonia and skin cancer.

Practising safe sex and avoiding direct contact with blood or blood products can reduce the risk of HIV infection. There is an extremely slight risk of acquiring HIV from contact on the sporting field with an HIV carrier who is bleeding or from bloodstained clothing. Attention to the SMA *Infectious Diseases Guidelines* will reduce this risk. Sports trainers managing bleeding athletes must stop the bleeding and remove all exposed blood. If bleeding cannot be controlled, the athlete should be removed from the field. Sports trainers should always wear gloves when managing an injury involving blood.

Sports Medicine Australia distributes an *Infectious Diseases Policy* and *Blood Rules OK* package that outlines recommendations for reducing the risk of transmitting infectious diseases. Copies are available from the SMA national office or your state/territory branch and can also be downloaded from the website at www.sma.org.au.

Glandular fever

Glandular fever occurs as a result of infection with the Epstein-Barr virus (EBV). The highest incidences of glandular fever are seen in adolescents and young adults.

SIGNS OF GLANDULAR FEVER

- Flu-like signs
- Fatigue
- Enlarged glands
- May develop a rash, depending on the medication being taken
- May have mild jaundice

SYMPTOMS OF GLANDULAR FEVER

- Flu-like symptoms
- Fever
- Sore throat

Older athletes have an increased tendency to develop complications such as hepatitis or a reduced platelet count (thrombocytopenia).

The incubation period can vary considerably but symptoms usually occur 4–6 weeks after infection with the virus. People with glandular fever can remain infectious for over a year even if their symptoms have settled completely.

MANAGEMENT OF GLANDULAR FEVER

Any athlete suspected of suffering from glandular fever should be referred to a doctor for assessment and management, usually including:

- resting from sporting activity until all acute symptoms have subsided
- avoiding contact sports if the spleen is enlarged
- treatment to reduce the fever and sore throat
- medical clearance before returning to competition and training.

Glandular fever is not particularly contagious despite the relatively high incidence in adolescents and young adults. There is no need for isolation of the athlete with glandular fever as most people have adequate antibody levels as a result of childhood exposure.

Chronic illness and injuries

Chronic illnesses, such as chronic asthma, are often well known to the athlete and sports trainer. They may present in a striking fashion, such as an epileptic seizure, or may appear in a subtle fashion in adulthood, such as adult-onset diabetes or leukaemia presenting as persistent tiredness.

The sports trainer should be alert to the athlete who looks unwell or 'off colour', particularly if this persists beyond 1 month. Referral to a doctor is the most important step in obtaining a diagnosis for the athlete.

Anaemia

Anaemia is the term used to describe insufficient red blood cells, which results in impaired oxygen-carrying capacity. It will affect performance in aerobic activity because of the impaired oxygen-carrying capacity of the blood. Anaemia needs medical attention and dietary support.

Anaemia can result in the athlete from intense sporting activity and is most common in female athletes usually because of blood loss related to menstruation.

Insufficient dietary iron will increase the risk of developing iron-deficiency anaemia. Anaemia can occur from other abnormalities in the biochemical pathways of red blood cell manufacture. These are generally related to non-absorption of particular essential nutrients, such as vitamin B12.

SIGNS OF ANAEMIA
- Pale skin
- Reduced sporting performance

SYMPTOMS OF ANAEMIA
- Tiredness
- Lethargy
- Shortness of breath

MANAGEMENT OF ANAEMIA

Iron deficiency should be suspected if an athlete complains of tiredness and their performance is impaired. It is particularly prevalent in vegetarians and female athletes during menstruation. The athlete should be referred to a doctor for assessment and management.

Osteoarthritis

Osteoarthritis is characterised by damage to the joints, particularly at the cartilage-covered articulating surfaces. It occurs from a combination of hereditary and environmental factors. Some sports will aggravate osteoarthritis of certain joints and are not recommended. Contact sports such as the football codes and prolonged weight-bearing sports such as long-distance running may be associated with the deterioration of hip and knee joints.

SIGNS OF OSTEOARTHRITIS
- Reduced distance the athlete is able to walk
- 'Clicking' of a joint
- Awkward movement at a joint

SYMPTOMS OF OSTEOARTHRITIS
- Pain at rest and during sleep may develop as the condition worsens
- Joint pain
- Stiffness after inactivity

MANAGEMENT OF OSTEOARTHRITIS

Although there is no treatment that can reverse the effects of osteoarthritis, it is important that athletes with this condition keep the surrounding muscle and bone in good condition and aim to achieve a normal range of motion at the affected joint. Non-weight bearing sports such as cycling, swimming and water polo are encouraged. Activities with a flexibility component, such as yoga, can be helpful in maintaining the range of motion as long as ligament instability is not an underlying cause of the osteoarthritis (e.g. in the knee).

A significant problem for athletes with osteoarthritis is that the pain of the condition can prevent them from being active, which causes weight gain that can in turn further aggravate their osteoarthritis. Non-weight-bearing activities such as those mentioned above can help prevent this cycle.

Glucosamine sulfate (with chondroitin sulfate) is an emerging therapeutic option for treating and preventing osteoarthritis. It has been shown to be effective in easing osteoarthritis pain in many people. It has potential benefits in rehabilitating cartilage, renewing synovial fluid and repairing joints that have been damaged from osteoarthritis.

Rheumatoid arthritis

Rheumatoid arthritis is a chronic condition that affects various body systems, particularly the peripheral joints, in a symmetrical pattern. The main feature of the disease is the persistent inflammation of the synovial lining of a joint, which leads to damage to the articular cartilage and the bone surrounding the joint. Eventually, joint deformity may occur.

The severity of rheumatoid arthritis varies from the occasional individual who has a short period of symptoms in one joint to those who have severe unremitting disease in multiple joints. Most people with rheumatoid arthritis have a complaint somewhere between these extremes.

The level of function permitted depends on the examination findings. The doctor examines the athlete for:

- functional capacity (ability to walk, run etc)
- joint swelling
- range of joint movement
- evidence of swelling of the affected joints.

This allows the rheumatoid arthritis to be categorised by the doctor as active or inactive. When the disease is inactive, with complete functional recovery, moderate to vigorous activity is allowed. If the disease is inactive but there is mild joint deterioration, gentle activity such as swimming is allowed. A good guide is what the athletes indicate they can tolerate in the way of physical activity.

It is important that the doctor responsible for the exercise program is able to observe the athlete exercising. It is impossible to predict how each individual will respond to a program without reviewing them at least regularly in the office, and hopefully in the field. The sports trainer is in a good position to report on how he or she sees the athlete coping with their activity; for example:

- Is the athlete limping more?
- Does the athlete appear to be in discomfort?

Chapter Nine

MOVING INJURED ATHLETES

LEARNING OUTCOMES

Demonstrate a sound knowledge and safe application of moving an injured athlete.

1   Demonstrate a range of transport techniques for injured athletes.
2   List appropriate precautions to be taken when transporting injured athletes.

ASSESSMENT OF OUTCOMES

Underpinning knowledge

You may be asked a number of written or oral questions related to the precautions for transporting injured athletes. You may also be asked to complete an online task or workbook with related activities.

Practical demonstration

You will be asked to demonstrate effective and safe transport of an injured athlete.

Scenario

You may be asked to transport a number of injured athletes in a simulated sporting environment.

Introduction

In the absence of expert medical help, moving an injured athlete should only be attempted when the athlete is in immediate danger or is capable of being moved safely. Sports trainers are often asked to make this judgement, which varies greatly from the expectations of a first aider. If the athlete is to be moved, it is important to select an appropriate method of movement for the safety of the athlete and the sports trainer.

There are several matters a sports trainer must consider before moving an injured athlete. They include:

- danger and safety
- location
- route of movement
- equipment
- personnel
- urgency
- lifting and carrying technique.

When a sports trainer might consider moving an injured athlete

Sports trainers are often expected to make rapid on-field assessments of an athlete's condition. Based on this assessment and the sports trainer's knowledge of sports medicine and first aid principles, there may be occasions when moving an athlete is appropriate. Some of these occasions may include:

- Hard or soft tissue injuries of the arm or hand when the sports trainer can provide adequate injury support during movement off the field.
- Soft tissue injuries of the leg, ankle or foot if the sports trainer can provide adequate support to the injury during movement. Stretchers and support staff should preferably be used. Hard tissue injuries of the lower limbs require appropriate splinting and a stretcher before moving the athlete.
- Most mild to moderate external bleeding injuries.
- Temperature-related illness or injury. Often athletes will need to be transported to a safer environment with less extreme temperature as part of their management.

Methods of moving an injured athlete

A sports trainer would have covered many types of casualty lifts and carries without equipment in their first aid training. In this chapter, we focus on some more advanced casualty moving techniques and

equipment available to sports trainers for moving injured athletes.

Moving athletes with suspected spinal injuries

An athlete with a suspected spinal injury should not be moved unless under the supervision of an experienced rescuer and/or paramedic with specific equipment. When moving such athletes, the priorities are:

- airway and circulation
- minimising movement of the head and cervical spine
- minimising movement of the thoracic and lumbar spine, sacrum and coccyx.

The athlete should be moved the shortest possible distance to a safe position. At all stages of the move, the body should be controlled in such a way that the head, neck and spine are immobilised as one body part. The athlete's arms and legs should first be moved closer to the trunk. Arms should be placed above the head or alongside the body to assist with efforts to roll the athlete like a log. Ideally, the athlete should be fitted with a cervical collar and placed on a spinal board or scoop stretcher.

Transporting athletes with spinal injuries

All athletes with a suspected spinal injury should be transported to hospital for further medical examination. Trained personnel should transport these injured athletes.

Athletes should only be transported if the following criteria have been met:

- DRSABCD principles have been checked.
- A cervical collar has been applied.
- A spinal board with straps has been applied.
- The head has been immobilised.

The athlete should be transported in the horizontal position with the appropriate number of first aiders assisting in the transportation. However, this may not be possible in all circumstances due to irregular terrain or obstacles.

Scoop stretchers, spine boards and cervical collars

An advantage of scoop stretchers is that they are assembled underneath the athlete without having to move them. Scoop stretchers can be used for any injury requiring minimal movement of an athlete. For suspected spinal injuries, a spine board can be used instead of a scoop stretcher.

In the case of a suspected spinal injury, a hard cervical collar should be fitted before moving the athlete with a scoop stretcher or spinal board. A cervical collar, which is designed to assist in maintaining the cervical spine in a neutral position, helps to minimise movement and the risk of further injury to the spinal cord.

Adjustable hard collars are the most suitable for sports situations as they take into account different body shapes and sizes. Sports trainers trained to fit a cervical collar must do so with the utmost care. If a sports trainer does not feel extremely confident in the application of a cervical collar, they should maintain manual head and neck immobilisation and wait for trained personnel to fit the device.

Stabilisation and transport of an athlete with a suspected spinal injury

In athletes with a suspected spinal injury, all due care should be taken to limit the movement of the spine while continuing to monitor and manage the airway. However, management of the airway takes precedence over management of the spinal injury.

A minimum of seven people is required to safely move an athlete with a suspected spinal injury.

USE OF SCOOP STRETCHERS

To safely move the injured athlete using a scoop stretcher, the following sequence should be adhered to:

1 The main operator should maintain and support the head in the neutral position by placing their hands on either side of the athlete's head. Ensure the head is maintained in the neutral position whenever possible.

2 Lay the stretcher beside the athlete and adjust it for the athlete's height.

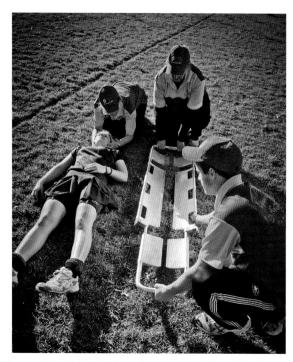

Figure 9.1 Maintain head support while adjusting scoop for athlete height

3 Detach both ends of the stretcher.

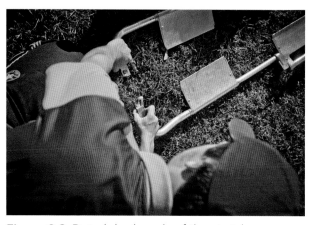

Figure 9.2 Detach both ends of the stretcher

4 Before fitting a cervical collar, ascertain the 'key dimension', which determines the size of the cervical collar to use for the athlete. The key dimension is the distance from the top of the athlete's shoulder to the bottom of the chin.

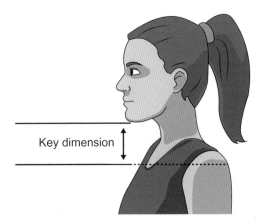

Figure 9.3 Key dimension for collar adjustment

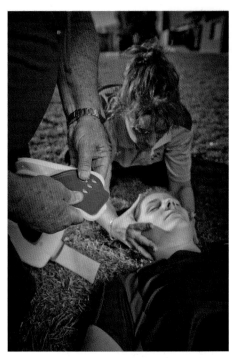

Figure 9.5 Adjusting a cervical collar to the key dimension

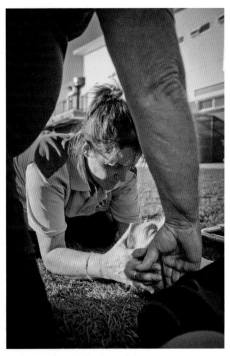

Figure 9.4 Measuring the key dimension

6 Gently slide the collar under the athlete's neck, being careful to ensure that there is no pressure placed on the trachea. The collar should be slid under the back of the neck with the velcro strip folded back.

7 Pass the strap underneath the athlete's neck and secure it in position with the velcro fasteners.

5 Select or adjust the cervical collar to fit the key dimension measurement.

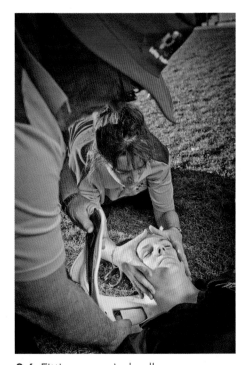

Figure 9.6 Fitting a cervical collar

8   Ensure that the collar has been fitted in the neutral position and is a snug fit around the neck, preventing movement.

9   Monitor the athlete constantly while continuing with spinal management.

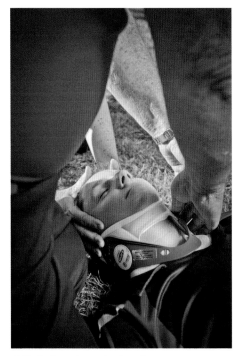

Figure 9.7 A fitted cervical collar

10 Slide both halves of the stretcher underneath the athlete and reattach both ends. The head end should be reattached first so the person at this end can stabilise the head while another person reattaches the foot end.

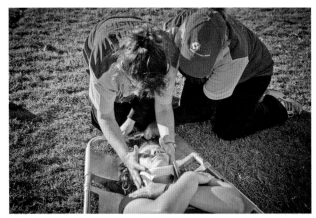

Figure 9.8 Maintain stabilisation of the head while reattaching the stretcher ends

11 When the athlete is ready to be moved, use appropriate lifting techniques to ensure no injury is caused to the lifters.

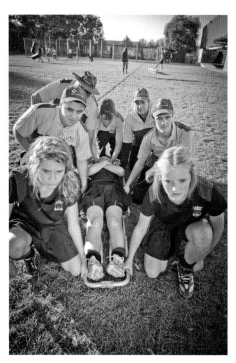

Figure 9.9 Use a safe lifting technique

USE OF SPINAL BOARDS

Spinal boards are rectangular and are hard and rigid, with handles along the side. They are designed to stabilise the spine and head in a neutral position. Most spinal boards have body straps attached for immobilisation and the facility to attach some form of head immobilisation. In most cases the sports trainer assists emergency medical personnel in the use of a spinal board.

The following steps apply to spinal board immobilisation in conscious or horizontal athletes.

1   If possible, maintain and support the head in the neutral position by placing your hands on either side of the athlete's head.

2   Trained personnel and trained sports trainers should only apply a cervical collar if they feel confident in doing so in accordance with the instructions in the section above.

3   Depending on the circumstances, highly trained first aiders may need to move the athlete (with minimal movement to the spine) so that a spinal board may be used.

4   With assistance, roll the athlete onto their side using a log roll while ensuring that the head and spine remain in a neutral position.

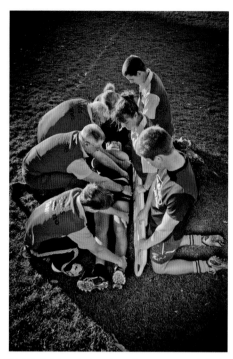

Figure 9.10 Maintaining head support while log rolling onto a spinal board

5 Gently position the spinal board against the athlete's back in line with their spine, ensuring the neutral position is maintained.

6 With the spinal board remaining as close to the back as possible at all times, slowly roll the athlete (and spinal board) backwards so that the spinal board ends up lying flat underneath the athlete's back in a horizontal position.

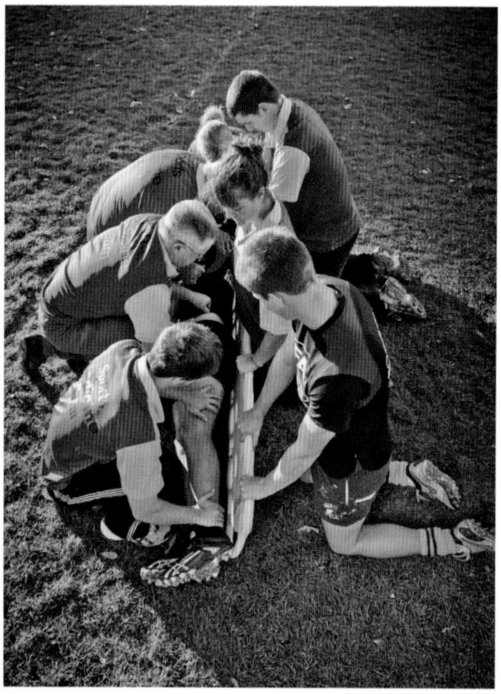

7 Secure and immobilise the athlete using head blocks or sand bags and fasten casualty straps around the body.

8 Offer constant reassurance to the athlete during this process and keep them informed as to what you are doing to prevent feelings of panic, which may cause the athlete to move.

9 Monitor the athlete's vital signs and condition until medical help arrives.

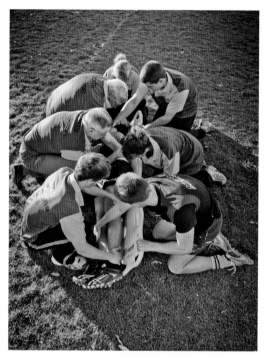

Figure 9.12 Personnel inserting arms to assist with the lowering of the patient

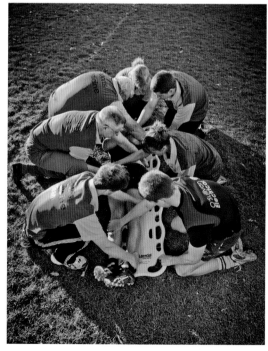

Figure 9.11 Keep the spine straight when rolling the athlete

Figure 9.13 Lower the patient to the ground, maintaining a straight spine

OTHER GRIPS FOR CERVICAL STABILISATION

In the absence of a suitable cervical collar, manual spinal immbolisation may be necessary. Two commonly used grips are the trapezius grip and the vice grip.

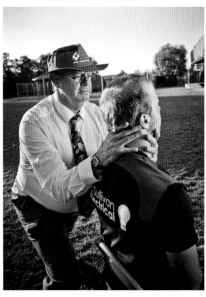

Figure 9.15 Vice grip in upright position

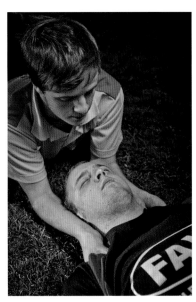

Figure 9.14 Trapezius grip

Chapter Ten

SPORTS TAPING

LEARNING OUTCOMES

Correctly apply sports-taping knowledge and procedures of joints that are commonly injured during sport.

1   List contraindications and precautions for taping.
2   Demonstrate effective preventive taping of an ankle.
3   Demonstrate effective preventive taping of a thumb.
4   Demonstrate effective taping of fingers.
5   Demonstrate the safe removal of tape from an athlete.
6   For Level 2 Sports Trainers, demonstrate the application of effective preventive taping of the knee and shoulder.

ASSESSMENT OF OUTCOMES

Underpinning knowledge

You may be asked a number of written or oral questions related to precautions and contraindications for sports taping. You may also be asked to complete an online task or workbook with related activities.

Practical demonstration

You will be asked to demonstrate effective preventive taping of an athlete's ankle, thumb and fingers. For the Level 2 Sports Trainer course, you will also be asked to demonstrate preventive taping for the knee and shoulder joints.

You will be asked to demonstrate the safe removal of tape from an athlete.

Scenario

You may be asked to perform preventive taping of a number of athletes in a simulated sporting environment.

Introduction

Taping is a skill commonly used by sports trainers to prevent injury and reduce the severity of injury. It involves the application of non-elastic (rigid) or elastic adhesive tape to restrict the range of movement at a particular joint. Historically, taping has been an important part of the sports trainer's role. Sports trainers must be proficient in this area of expertise at all times.

Aims of taping

The aim of taping is to:

- prevent injury
- limit further injury
- provide support
- limit pain
- limit specific movements at a joint
- allow desired movements at a joint.

Taping a joint to prevent injury should not replace a strengthening or rehabilitation program. Tape provides additional support only; it cannot replace the stability provided by natural structures. Thus, if an injury or joint weakness is present a rehabilitation program provided by a health professional is necessary.

Only trained personnel, such as a sports trainer or physiotherapist, should apply adhesive tape. Taping that is applied incorrectly may aggravate an existing injury or cause a new injury.

Materials

Adhesive tape

Modern adhesive tapes can be non-elastic (rigid) or elastic and have a number of qualities that make them suitable for use in sport and for treatment of sports injuries. They possess a uniform adhesive mass and relative strength and are lightweight. All these qualities are of value in supporting injured joints and holding wound dressings in place.

TAPE GRADE

Rigid adhesive tape is often graded according to the number of longitudinal and vertical fibres per centimetre of backing material. The heavier and more expensive tapes contain more strengthening fibres than the lighter and less expensive tapes. However, a lighter tape may prove more suitable for those athletes with sensitive skin.

RIGID ADHESIVE TAPE

Rigid adhesive tape is the most commonly used tape for prevention of injury. This tape is available in a variety of widths, such as 12 mm, 25 mm, 38 mm and 50 mm. It is important for the correct size to be used for each specific taping procedure.

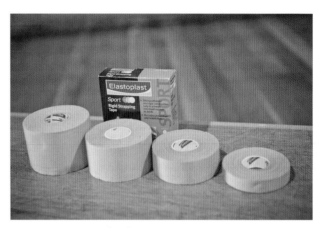

Figure 10.1 Rigid adhesive tape

ELASTIC ADHESIVE TAPE

Elastic adhesive tape is also sometimes used in sports medicine. Elastic adhesive tape stretches and readily conforms to uneven surfaces. There are many different products sold under different names and with differing claimed or intended benefits. Some forms of elastic adhesive tape are not intended to limit joint movement in the same way as rigid sports tape; they use the elastic properties of the tape to assist muscle activity or stimulate some other physiological processes. Other types of elastic adhesive tape can be used for holding dressings in place and covering tape/dressings on irregularly shaped surfaces. Elastic adhesive tape is available in a variety of thicknesses and with widths ranging from 15 to 100 mm.

Care should be taken not to apply elastic adhesive tape too tightly as it can impair circulation; it should not be used on joints to restrict the range of motion due to the risk of it being applied too tightly.

Rigid adhesive tape prevents ankle, thumb and finger sprains more effectively than elastic adhesive tape when used correctly.

Tape storage

When storing tape, a sports trainer must ensure that it is:

- stored in a cool place (such as a low cupboard)
- stacked so that it rests on its flat side so that it does not become distorted.

Tape characteristics

All adhesive tape should:
- maintain its adherence to the skin despite perspiration and activity
- contain as few skin irritants as possible
- be able to be removed without leaving a residue on the skin or pulling away the skin.

Tape selection

Adhesive tape should be selected according to:
- the size of the athlete
- the size of the joint being taped
  - narrower tape is better for smaller joints such as fingers and thumbs
  - wider tape is better for large joints such as the ankle and shoulder
- the duration and type of activity.

Associated materials that may assist taping

Elastic under-wrap

Some athletes may be allergic or sensitive to the adhesive on the tape. Always ask the athlete if they have used tape before and if they reacted to it. If this is the case and the athlete wants to proceed with the taping, gain consent and cover the area to be taped with an elastic under-wrap.

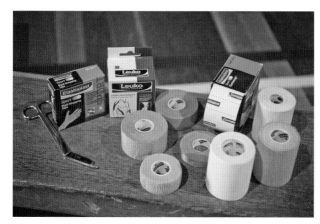

Figure 10.2 Tapes and associated materials

To enhance the effectiveness of taping over under-wrap:
- the area must be free of body hair
- if gauze pads are to be used, apply them as described in the section below.

Using under-wrap can reduce the effectiveness of the taping.

Gauze pads

Areas where the skin is loose to allow movement are susceptible to cuts from tape. The most commonly cut areas are over the Achilles tendon and across the anterior aspect of the ankle joint. A small amount of petroleum jelly and then a gauze pad can be applied to these areas prior to taping to prevent tape cuts. If there is a tape cut or any other skin injury in the area to be taped, it is essential that the wound be covered with gauze pads prior to taping.

Cushioning foam

Foam may be used to prevent blisters or to cushion tender areas due to large bumps (protuberances), such as the malleoli on each side of the ankle joint. When applying foam, cut a horseshoe or doughnut-shaped ring and place it over the bump to take the pressure off the highest point.

Tape adhesive

Spray-on tape adhesive is often used to ensure the tape is effective, especially when the athlete sweats or is likely to get wet. Use it with caution as it often has a strong odour and can be toxic if inhaled.

Tape remover

Tape remover is a spray-on or soaking solution that allows tape to be removed easily.

Using adhesive tape for sports injuries

When using adhesive tape for sports injuries, the main considerations for sports trainers are:
- preparation for taping
- appropriate positioning of the athlete for the body area to be taped
- the proper application and method of taping
- tearing the adhesive tape
- post-taping checks and warning the athlete regarding precautions
- removing the tape.

Preparation for taping

Applying adhesive tape directly onto the skin provides maximum support. To provide maximum support to the athlete, ensure:
- the application area is clean and dry with no dirt, oil or lotions
- hair has been removed from the application area at least 12 hours prior to taping if possible
- padding has been applied to areas that require protection
- tape is only applied when the application area is at normal body temperature
- a tape adhesive is applied if additional adhesion is required

- under-wrap is applied if the athlete is allergic or sensitive to the adhesive on the tape
- the area is free of body hair when applying under-wrap and tape adhesive is used prior to applying it.

Appropriate positioning of the athlete for the body area to be taped

For the best possible application of tape, it is important to ensure the body area to be taped is placed in an optimal position to enable the required movement or restrict it, as applicable. The athlete needs to be positioned so that they are safe and comfortable. They should be encouraged to maintain their position during the taping application as movement of the area being taped may render the taping technique ineffective.

Proper application and method of taping

There are many considerations and opinions on the best taping technique. It is, however, important to consider the following in all instances:

- Select appropriate sized tape for the area and for the degree of restriction of movement required.
- Place the joint in the appropriate position to achieve your objective.
- If taping over a muscle, allow for contraction and expansion of the area.
- Avoid continuous taping. Make one circle at a time to prevent constriction.
- Overlap the tape by a half to a third of the width of the tape below.
- Tape from the roll whenever possible. Tape laid from the roll will conform to the area better and your speed, proficiency and efficiency will be improved.
- When taping from the roll, ensure the tape is laid on and smoothed out and not pulled too tightly.
- Allow the tape to fit the contours of the area. Rigid tape will not bend around acute angles. Do not allow wrinkles or gaps as they will irritate or cut the skin.
- Start taping with an 'anchor' piece. The anchor provides a stable base for the strips that follow.
- Finish with a 'lock' piece. The lock ensures the supporting strips will not peel away during activity.

Tearing adhesive tape

Sports trainers use a variety of different methods for tearing adhesive tape. Whichever method is used,

the sports trainer should be able to keep the tape roll in their hand most of the time. The following is a suggested procedure:

1 Hold the tape roll in the preferred hand with the index finger pressing its outer edge.
2 With the other hand, grasp the loose end between the thumb and the index finger.
3 With both hands in place, pull both ends of the tape so that it is tight.
4 Next, make a quick, scissor-like move to tear the tape. In tearing tape, the movement of one hand is away from the body and that of the other hand is towards the body. Do not try to twist or bend the tape in attempting to tear it.

Some people do not possess the strength or skill to tear tape effectively or the tape may be too rigid to tear manually. In this case, using a knife, scissors or razor blade may be warranted. Ensure such items are used with care around athletes to prevent unnecessary injury.

Learning to tear adhesive tape effectively from many different positions is essential for speed and efficiency.

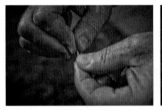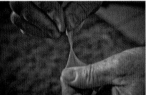

Figure 10.3 Correct manual tearing of tape

Post-taping checks

In order for a sports trainer to confirm that the taping they have carried out is effective and safe, the following checks should be undertaken:

- Check for impaired circulation (capillary refill):
  - Lightly press the skin distal to the tape – normal colour should rapidly reappear.
- Check for impaired sensation:
  - Does the athlete have pins and needles or numbness?
  - Can the athlete feel the area?
  - Is there any pain?
  - Does the tape feel too tight?
- Check that the taping limits the movements it was intended to limit:
  - Get the athlete to move the joint in various ways and ensure the movement is limited in the desired directions.

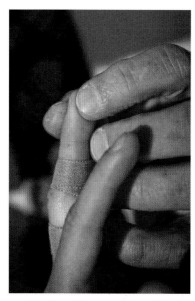

Figure 10.4 Checking for capillary refill

Removing tape

Tape can usually be removed from the skin by hand or using scissors or a chemical adhesive solvent.

MANUAL REMOVAL

1 Soak the tape in tape remover or some other safe adhesive solvent.

2 Do not wrench the tape from the skin.

3 Pull the tape back on itself and place pressure on the skin as close as possible to the line of attachment to the tape.

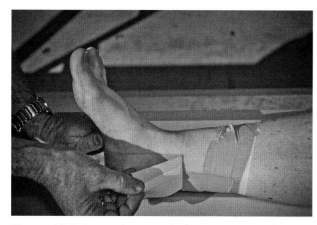

Figure 10.5 Manual removal of tape

SCISSORS OR TAPE CUTTERS

When using scissors or tape cutters, ensure the blunt nose is under the tape.

CHEMICAL ADHESIVE SOLVENTS

Use only medically approved adhesive solvents. Many industrial or commercial solvents may be toxic.

Taping of the hand (fingers and thumb)

The hand is commonly injured during sporting activity. It is important that the sports trainer has a good understanding of the anatomy and functioning of the hand in order to effectively manage injuries.

Bones of the hand

The hand consists of:

- carpal bones (wrist)
- metacarpal bones (hand)
- phalanges (fingers and thumb).

There are eight carpal bones, arranged in two rows of four. The proximal row of carpals meets with the radius and ulna. The distal row moves (articulates) with the five metacarpal bones that form the palm of the hand. The metacarpals move (articulate) proximally with the bones that form the fingers (phalanges).

The fingers consist of three bones, called the proximal phalanx, middle phalanx and distal phalanx. The thumb has only two bones, the proximal phalanx and distal phalanx.

Joints and ligaments of the hand

The joint between two phalanges is called an interphalangeal joint. Flexion and extension are the only movements at this joint.

The joint between the metacarpal and proximal phalanx is referred to as the metacarpophalangeal joint. Flexion and extension with some abduction and adduction occur at this joint.

In the hand, the proximal end of the first metacarpal bone and a carpal bone meet to create the first carpometacarpal joint. Circumduction and opposition movements can occur at this joint, allowing the thumb to rotate about its long axis and pick up objects along with the fingers.

The interphalangeal and metacarpophalangeal joints both have:

- articular capsules
- palmar ligaments (medial)
- collateral ligaments (lateral)
- volar place ligaments on the anterior (palm side) of the thumb that prevent hyperextension.

Muscles of the hand

There are many muscles that control the movements of the thumb and fingers. The sports trainer should be aware of the following groups.

THUMB MUSCLES

- Flexors of the thumb
- Extensors of the thumb
- Abductors of the thumb
- Adductors of the thumb

- Opponents of the thumb (the action of bringing the thumb opposite to the fingers)

FINGER MUSCLES

- Flexors of the fingers
- Extensors of the fingers

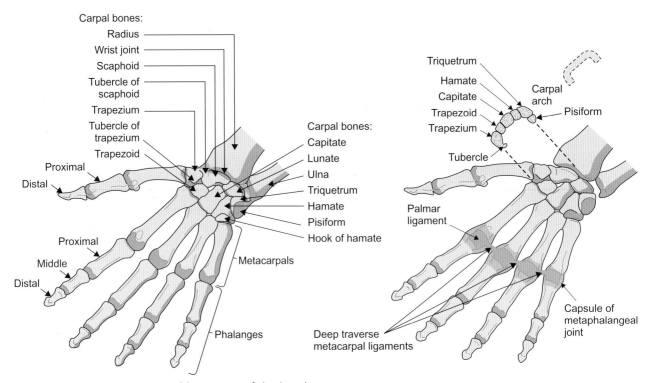

Figure 10.6 Bones, joints and ligaments of the hand

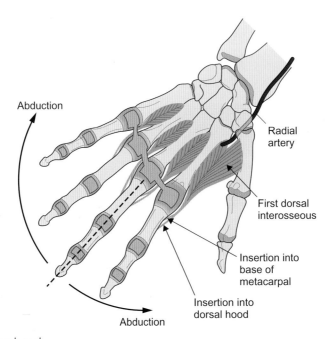

Figure 10.7 Muscles of the hand

Considerations when taping fingers and thumbs

Fingers and thumbs that have been weakened by jarring or a sprain may require protection from more serious injury. The application of rigid tape may provide the necessary additional support.

The joints surrounding the fingers and the thumb can be easily dislocated and seriously damaged by incorrect taping technique. When taping these joints, consider the following:

- the range of movement at the particular joint being taped
- the structure you are trying to support.

Narrow, rigid adhesive tape is usually preferable for the finger and thumb techniques. Alternatively, 38 mm rigid adhesive tape may be ripped into narrow strips and used instead.

Taping fingers

The fingers are commonly injured in sport because they are constantly exposed to risk.

Fingers are taped:

- for anatomical splinting as a part of initial management
- for protection of an injured finger during rehabilitation
- to prevent re-injury.

With new (acute) injuries, it is rarely necessary to splint injured fingers. If such splinting is necessary, only a doctor or physiotherapist should perform it. Buddy-taping will adequately manage most finger injuries.

TECHNIQUE FOR BUDDY-TAPING FINGERS

1 Ensure the fingers are clean and dry.
2 Pad between the fingers with a small piece of gauze or soft splint.
3 Tape two adjacent fingers together.
4 Tape above and below the injured joint.

Check:

- Distal capillary refill
- Movement and sensation
- Restriction

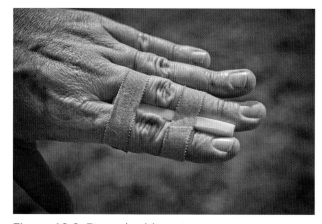

Figure 10.8 Finger buddy-taping

Taping thumbs

The thumb is commonly injured in sport. The anatomy of the thumb is very complex. It has great mobility, which increases the risk of injury occurring.

Hyperextension injuries often occur and may cause ligament damage or fractures.

The aim of taping the thumb is to:

- prevent injury
- decrease the severity of the injury if an injury does occur.

TECHNIQUE FOR TAPING A THUMB

1 Apply an anchor strip around the wrist.
2 For extra support, apply strips of tape from the distal thumb anchor to the wrist anchor. These strips create a fan pattern and should be anchored around the distal thumb and around the wrist.
3 Take the tape from the medial side of the wrist diagonally across the back of the hand, aiming for the base of the thumb.
4 Gently encircle the tape around the proximal phalanx of the thumb.
5 Form a second circle as close to the base of the thumb as possible.
6 On completion of the second circle the tape crosses the back of the metacarpophalangeal joint, forming a cross with the original diagonal strip.
7 Continue the tape diagonally across the soft pad of the muscle on the palm side of the base of the thumb.
8 Encircle the wrist for the final time.

Check:

- Distal capillary refill
- Movement and sensation
- Restriction

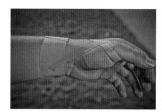 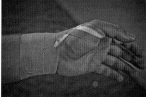

Figure 10.9 Thumb-taping sequence

Taping of the ankle

The ankle is probably the most commonly sprained joint during sporting activity. It is important for the sports trainer to have a good understanding of the anatomy and functioning of the ankle to manage injuries effectively.

Bones of the ankle

The ankle is essentially a type of twin-hinge joint formed by the movement (articulation) of three bones.

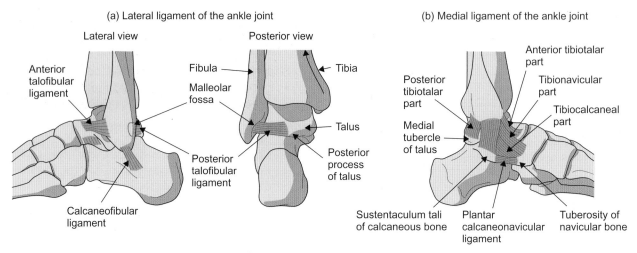

Figure 10.10 Bones, joint and ligaments of the ankle

The three bones of the ankle joint are:

- the tibia and the fibula, which form a socket at the lower end of the leg
- the talus, which fits into this socket. The talus is wedge-shaped so that the ankle is firmly locked when dorsiflexed. On plantar flexion, the talus is relatively loose in its socket.

The heel bone (calcaneus) is the weight-bearing bone of the ankle joint. It is closely attached to the talus by ligaments allowing it to act as an extension of the talus. If excessive movements of the calcaneus can be controlled, excessive movements of the talus will also be controlled. This is important when taping the ankle.

Joint and ligaments of the ankle

The four directions of movement at the ankle are:

- plantar flexion – occurs at the true ankle joint between the talus and tibia and fibula
- dorsiflexion – occurs at the true ankle joint between the talus and tibia and fibula
- inversion – occurs at joints distal to the true ankle joint
- eversion – occurs at joints distal to the true ankle joint.

The medial ligaments at the ankle joint are strong and attach to the medial side of the tibia and the calcaneus. These ligaments prevent eversion at the ankle joint. The lateral ligaments of the ankle joint are composed of three slim ligaments that attach the fibula to the talus and the calcaneus. These ligaments prevent inversion at the ankle joint. The medial and lateral ligaments also help to prevent the talus from sliding forwards out of its joint.

Muscles of the ankle

There are muscles that travel from the lower leg down to the ankle. The tendons of these muscles pass over the anterior surface of the ankle joint and behind the medial and lateral malleoli. These muscles require regular exercise to maintain their strength so they can help the ligaments support the ankle joint.

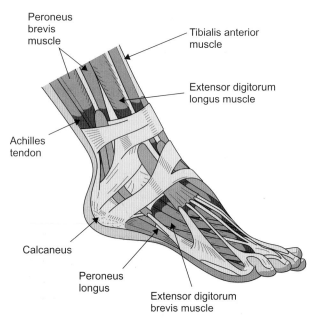

Figure 10.11 Muscles of the ankle

Taping an ankle

Ankle taping applied directly to the athlete's skin affords the greatest support.

The aim of taping an ankle is to:

- provide protection
- prevent injury
- decrease the severity of the injury if an injury does occur.

TECHNIQUE FOR TAPING AN ANKLE

1 Ensure the ankle and lower leg are clean and dry.
2 Position the foot at 90°.
3 Apply protective padding and cover any existing wounds.
4 Apply two anchor strips around the base of the calf muscle:
   a the first strip at the base of the calf
   b the second strip overlapping the first by half the width of the tape.

Apply 2–3 stirrups (depending upon the size of the foot/ankle)

1 Begin from the anchor on the medial side, cover half the malleoli, hook underneath the heel and finish at the anchor on the lateral side.
2 The second and third stirrup should be applied as for the first stirrup but should overlap the first by half the width of the tape.

Apply a figure of 6

Begin from the anchor on the medial side, follow the stirrup under the heel and return across the front of the ankle to where the tape commenced.

Closing down of stirrups

1 Start above the ankle and work down the leg.
2 Apply separate strips of tape, each overlapping their predecessor by half the width of the tape until the stirrups are covered.
3 Finish at the malleoli (bony part of the ankle).

Heel locks (two complete sets)

1 Commence at the front of the ankle and lay the tape diagonally across the top of the foot towards the medial side of the calcaneus:
   a across the malleoli
   b around the back of the calcaneus
   c under the calcaneus
   d across the front of the foot.
2 Repeat this sequence from the lateral side.

Closing down

Lay a piece of tape gently around the midfoot, covering the extreme edges of the heel locks.
Check:
■ Distal capillary refill
■ Movement and sensation
■ Restriction

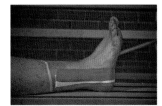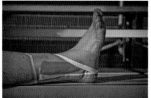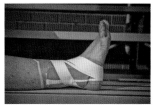

Figure 10.12 Ankle-taping sequence

Ankle bracing

Ankle bracing is an alternative to taping and has been shown to be a cost-effective method of preventing ankle sprains and reducing the severity of the injury. The ankle brace is worn inside the athlete's shoe and is usually laced or secured with velcro-type adhesive.

Advantages of bracing compared to taping:
■ Braces are easy and quick to use.
■ Braces are re-usable.
■ Braces may be cost-effective over the long term.
■ Braces can easily be retightened during a break in the game to regain effective ankle support.
■ Braces do not require skilled instructors.
■ There is less skin irritation due to allergies.

Disadvantages of bracing compared to taping:
■ The possibility the brace may slip during exercise.
■ The weight of the brace.
■ Sometimes it may be difficult to obtain the correct size.
■ It may wear out at an inconvenient time.
■ A custom-made brace may be necessary.

Studies regarding the effectiveness of braces during and after exercise are as controversial as are those for taping, with the results being varied and inconsistent. It has been shown that braces do provide additional support to the ankle, but the results as to whether they provide more support than taping are inconsistent.

Taping of the knee

The knee is one of the most commonly injured joints during sports. It is important for the sports trainer to have a good understanding of the anatomy and functioning of the knee joint in order to effectively manage injuries or prevent future injuries.

Bones of the knee

The main bones of the knee joint are the femur, the tibia, the patella (kneecap) and the fibula.

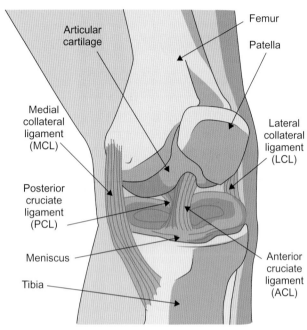

Figure 10.13 Bones, joints and ligaments of the knee

Joint and ligaments of the knee

The knee is a large hinge joint that primarily allows flexion and extension between the femur and tibia. The knee is reinforced by strong ligaments that are vulnerable to injury during sport.

Taping a knee

Knee taping applied directly to the athlete's skin affords the greatest support.

The aim of taping the knee is to:

- provide protection
- prevent injury
- decrease the severity of the injury if an injury does occur.

TECHNIQUE FOR TAPING A KNEE FOR A MEDIAL COLLATERAL LIGAMENT INJURY

1 Ensure the knee is clean and dry.

2 Position the athlete standing with the knee slightly bent and the heel placed on a roll of tape or a small block.

3 Apply protective padding and cover any existing wounds.

4 Apply two anchor strips approximately 10 cm above and below the knee joint while asking the athlete to contract the muscles underneath:

   a Place the superior anchor on the quadriceps muscles 10 cm above the knee joint.

   b Place the inferior anchor on the calf muscles 10 cm below the knee joint.

5 Apply a diagonal tape strip starting anteriorly on the inferior anchor and, while tensioning the tape, place it in a diagonal direction posteriorly on the superior anchor.

6 Apply a diagonal tape strip starting posteriorly on the inferior anchor and, while tensioning the tape, place it in a diagonal direction anteriorly on the superior anchor. The two diagonal tape strips should form an X over the medial collateral ligament of the knee.

7 Repeat steps 5 and 6 twice, with each pair of diagonal strips overlapping the previous pair by half the width of the tape. When completed, you should have 3 pairs of overlapping diagonals.

8 Reinforce this with up to 3 vertical strips of tape from the inferior anchor to the superior anchor and directly over the medial collateral ligament of the knee.

9 Apply 2 lock-off strips, one over the superior anchor and one over the inferior anchor, while asking the athlete to contract the muscles underneath once again.

10 If necessary, or if swelling is present, elastic adhesive tape may be applied over the taping for additional compression or to hold the tape in place during play.

Check:

- Distal capillary refill
- Movement and sensation
- Restriction

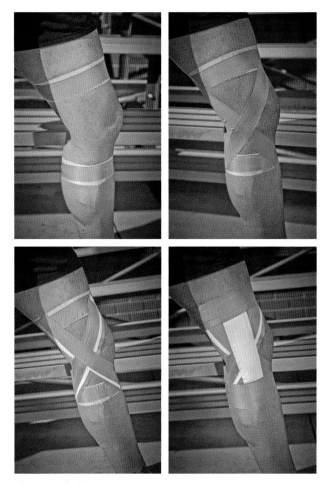

Figure 10.14 Knee-taping sequence

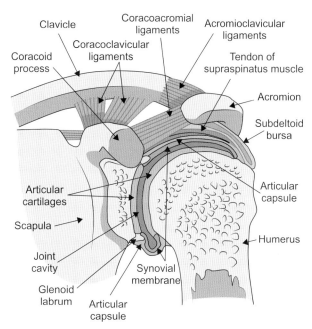

Figure 10.15 Bones, joints and ligaments of the shoulder

Taping of the shoulder

The shoulder joint is commonly injured during sports, with dislocation or subluxation of the joints or muscle/tendon tears and strains being the most prevalent injuries. It is important for the sports trainer to have a good understanding of the anatomy and functioning of the shoulder joint in order to effectively manage injuries or prevent future injuries.

Bones of the shoulder

The main bones making up the shoulder joint are the scapula, the clavicle (collarbone) and the humerus.

Joints and ligaments of the shoulder

The shoulder consists of the glenohumeral joint (between the scapula and the humerus) and the acromioclavicular joint (between the scapula and the clavicle).

Taping a shoulder

Shoulder taping applied directly to the athlete's skin affords the greatest support.

The aim of taping the shoulder is to:

- provide protection
- prevent injury
- decrease the severity of the injury if an injury does occur.

TECHNIQUE FOR TAPING A SHOULDER

1. Ensure the shoulder is clean and dry.
2. Position the athlete sitting with the hand placed on their waist so that the shoulder is in 45° abduction.
3. Apply a foam ring or hypoallergenic underlay around the nipple for protection.
4. If available, to protect the skin apply hypoallergenic underlay tape where the superior and inferior anchors are to be placed.
5. Apply a superior anchor on the trunk. Using a long vertical strip, start anteriorly below the nipple and tension the tape while directing it superiorly over the clavicle and down posteriorly on the scapula to the same length as the anterior portion of the tape. Ensure the tape is not pulled down over the clavicle

as this may cause discomfort and interfere with circulation and nerve function.

6 Apply a horizontal strip of tape under the axilla (armpit), joining together the ends of the anterior and posterior portions of the long vertical strip.

7 Apply a circumferential inferior anchor halfway on the upper arm (approximately 3 cm below the deltoid muscle insertion).

8 Apply a diagonal strip of tape, starting posteriorly on the inferior anchor on the arm and directing the tape diagonally and laterally over the upper arm (middle of the deltoid muscle), to place it anteriorly on the superior anchor strip at about 5 cm below the clavicle.

9 Apply a diagonal strip of tape, starting anteriorly on the inferior anchor on the arm and directing the tape diagonally and laterally over the upper arm (middle of the deltoid muscle), to place it posteriorly on the superior anchor strip at about 5 cm below the top of the shoulder. The diagonals should form an X over the lateral aspect of the arm (over the deltoid muscle).

10 Repeat steps 8 and 9 with two more pairs of tape diagonals, overlapping each pair by approximately half the width of the previous pair of tape diagonals. There should be 3 pairs of tape diagonals forming an X over the lateral aspect of the upper arm (middle of the deltoid muscle).

11 Apply 3 overlapping vertical strips on the lateral aspect of the arm, each starting on the lateral aspect of the inferior anchor and finishing at the middle of the superior anchor on the top of the shoulder.

12 Apply 2 lock-offs, one over the superior anchor and one over the inferior anchor, to ensure all tape strips are secured in place.

Check:

- Distal capillary refill
- Movement of the shoulder
- Sensation under the tape and in the arm and hand
- Restriction of required movement

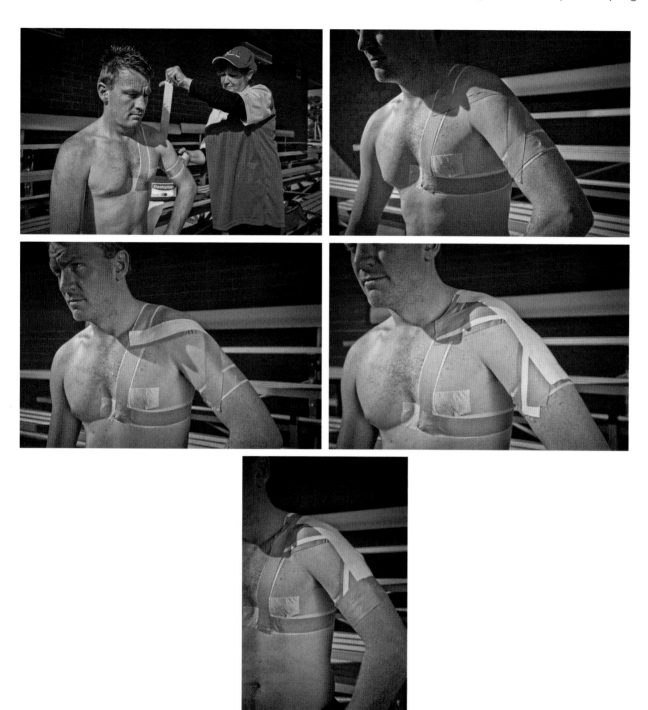

Figure 10.16 Shoulder-taping sequence

APPENDIX A
Sports first aid kit contents

Depending on state/territory and governing body regulations, Sports Medicine Australia recommends the following as minimum contents of a sports trainer's first aid supplies.

No.	Product	Used for
2	Gauze swabs 7.5 cm × 7.5 cm × 5 sets	Applying lotions and bathing of wounds
1	Thermal blanket/space blanket	Cover casualty – when cold or windy, or to treat shock
1	Premium sports tape 38 mm × 13.7 mm	Rigid strapping – suitable for taping ankle
10	Latex gloves	Hygiene
1	Plastic bag	Disposal of blood-soiled dressings
1	Orthopaedic support foam 10 cm × 15 cm	Can help stop blisters rubbing
1	Triangular bandage	Fracture immobilisation – sling
1	Cultiplast dressings adhesive 7.2 cm × 5.0 cm × 5 sets	Wound dressing – covering of minor cuts
1	Cultiplast dressings adhesive 10.0 cm × 8.0 cm × 5 sets	Wound dressing – covering of larger cuts
2	Tricose 5.0 cm × 5.0 cm (small) non-stick	Cover wound for protection of smaller wounds
2	Tricose 7.5 cm × 7.5 cm (large) non-stick	Cover wound for protection of larger wounds
2	Butterfly strips 6 mm × 76 mm	Wound closure strip (e.g. bring wound edges together)
2	Betadine swab sticks	Cleaning wound – antiseptic
1	First aid strips × 24 sets	Minor cuts/abrasions
2	Saline plastic ampoules	Eye irrigation/cleaning wound
1	Conforming gauze bandage 2.5 cm	Secures dressing in place – small wound
1	Conforming gauze bandage 5.0 cm	Secures dressing in place – medium wound
1	Conforming gauze bandage 7.5 cm	Secures dressing in place – large wound
2	Crepe bandages medium weight 7.5 cm	Wound cover – secures general purpose/light dressing in place
1	Crepe bandage heavy duty 7.5 cm	Compression strapping/support (ankle) Wound cover – secures dressing in place
1	Crepe bandage heavy duty 10.0 cm	Compression strapping/support (knee) Wound cover – secures dressing in place
1	Ventolin inhaler and spacer	Asthma attacks
1	Hypoallergenic adhesive tape	Secures dressing – ideal for sensitive skin
1	Betadine liquid	Wound cleaning antiseptic
1	Premium sports tape 2.5 cm × 2.5 cm	Stretch strapping – finger tape
1	Forceps, stainless steel	Tweezers for splinter removal – keep sterile
1	Scissors, stainless steel	Cut dressings and bandages
10	Disposable splinter probes	Discard after use – safely
1	Metsal cream 50 g	Relief from muscular pain (not to be used on a new soft tissue injury for the first 48 h) Used after **R**est **I**ce **C**ompression **E**levation **R**eferral

(Continued)

No.	Product	Used for
2	Cutinova Thin dressings 5.0 cm × 6.0 cm	Hydro (water) active wound dressing for blisters and open wounds (place directly over cuts for blood rule problems)
1	Handy tubular bandage size D	Knee/arm dressing – retains dressings in place and gives compression
1	Premium sports tape 2.5 cm × 5.0 m	Rigid strapping – strapping ankles
RECOMMENDED EXTRAS		
1	Resuscitation mask	To assist with EAR in CPR – sports trainer should have received training in use
1	Universal shears	Cutting dressings and clothing
1	Examination torch	
	Assorted sizes tubular bandage	Secure dressing on difficult areas
	Assorted sizes Surgifix net bandage	Secure dressing on high body movement areas
1	Sunscreen 30+	Protection from sun and ultraviolet rays
	Sports injury pack	Cold pack and compression bandage for initial treatment of soft tissue injuries. Rest Ice Compression Elevation Referral
1	Water bottle	Fluid replacement

APPENDIX B
Sports trainer management flow chart

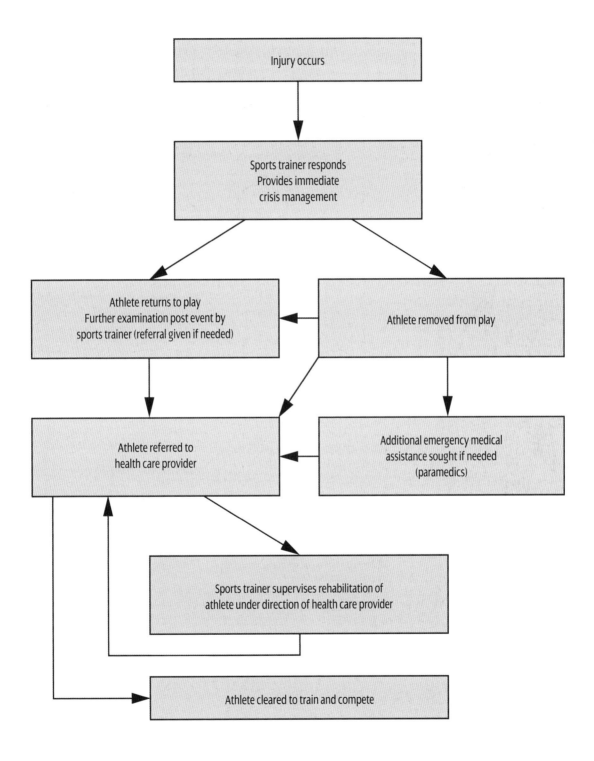

Injury occurs

Sports trainer responds
Provides immediate
crisis management

Athlete returns to play
Further examination post event by
sports trainer (referral given if needed)

Athlete removed from play

Athlete referred to
health care provider

Additional emergency medical
assistance sought if needed
(paramedics)

Sports trainer supervises rehabilitation of
athlete under direction of health care provider

Athlete cleared to train and compete

APPENDIX C

Injury report form

Sports Injury Reporting Form

SPORTS MEDICINE AUSTRALIA

Name: _____ Address: _____

Sport:_____ Event: _____ Venue: _____ Team: _____

Today's date: _____/_____/_____ Time _____:_____ am/pm   Gender: ❑ Male ❑ Female   Date of Birth: _____/_____/_____

Injured person (*please circle*): Player / Referee / Coach / Spectator

---

TYPE OF ACTIVITY AT TIME OF INJURY
❑ training
❑ warm-up
❑ competition
❑ cool-down
❑ other _____

REASON FOR PRESENTATION
❑ new injury
❑ aggravated injury
❑ recurrent injury
❑ illness
❑ other

BODY PARTS INJURED
circle and name

NATURE OF INJURY/ILLNESS
❑ bruise/contusion
❑ cardiac problem
❑ cold/flu
❑ concussion
❑ disclocation/subluxation
❑ fracture (including suspected)
❑ inflammation/swelling
❑ loss of consciousness
❑ overuse injury
❑ respiratory problem
❑ skin injury e.g. graze/cut/blisters
❑ sprain e.g. ligament tear
❑ strain e.g. muscle tear
❑ unspecifed medical condition
❑ other _____

CAUSE OF INJURY
❑ collision with fixed object
❑ collision with other player
❑ fall from height/awkward landing
❑ jumping to shoot or defend
❑ overexertion
❑ overuse
❑ slip/trip/fall/stumble
❑ struck by ball/object
❑ struck by other player
❑ temperature related
❑ other _____

Explain how the incident occured
_____
_____
_____
_____
_____
_____
_____

Were there any contributing factors to the incident? *e.g. unsuitable footwear, playing surface, equipment, foul play*
_____
_____
_____

Was protective equipment worn on the injured body part?
❑ Yes   ❑ No
If yes, what? e.g. mouthguard, brace?
_____
_____

INITIAL TREATMENT
❑ none given (not required)
❑ CPR
❑ dressing
❑ immobilisation
❑ RICER
❑ sling/splint
❑ strapping/taping
❑ stretch/exercises
❑ transport from field/court
❑ other _____

ADVICE GIVEN
❑ immediate return to activity
❑ return to play with restriction
_____
_____
❑ unable to return at present
❑ referred for further assessment before returning to activity

NOTICE
The injured person told that if injury/ illness does NOT improve in the following 24 hours they MUST seek further advice from their own medical professional.
❑ Yes   ❑ No

REFERRAL
❑ no referral
❑ medical practitioner
❑ physiotherapist
❑ ambulance
❑ hospital
❑ other _____

PROVISIONAL SEVERITY ASSESSMENT
❑ mild (1–7 days modified activity)
❑ moderate (8–21 days modified activity)
❑ severe (>21 days modified or lost)

TREATING PERSON
❑ Sports Trainer/Sports First Aider (ID _____)
❑ medical practitioner
❑ physiotherapist
❑ other _____

Signature of injured person

_____

Signature of treating person

_____

Date: _____/_____/_____

APPENDIX D

Athlete medical profile form

Athlete Medical Profile – Personal Record

All information on this sheet is confidential.
Access to this sheet is limited to Director, Sports First Aider, Sports Trainer and Coach.

Personal Details

Surname

Given Names

Address — Number — Street / Road

Suburb / Town / City — State — Postcode

Home Phone — Area Code — Number

Mobile / Business Phone — Number

Sex M ☐ F ☐   Date of Birth — Day / Month / Year   Age — Years   Height — Centimetres   Weight — Kilograms

Blood Group   Do you object to transfusions? Yes ☐ No ☐

Emergency Contact

Surname

Given Names

Home Phone — Area Code — Number

Mobile / Business Phone — Number

Relationship

Health Care Details

Medicare Number

Private Health Insurance Yes ☐ No ☐ Fund

Private Doctor

Telephone — Area Code — Number

Address — Number — Street / Road

Suburb / Town / City — State — Postcode

Can Doctor be contacted at all times? Yes ☐ No ☐

Private Dentist

Telephone — Area Code — Number

Address — Number — Street / Road

Suburb / Town / City — State — Postcode

Can Dentist be contacted in emergency? Yes ☐ No ☐

(Continued)

Current History

Current medical problems

Regular medications including supplements, stating name and dosage

Allergies

Sports injuries (Please list any injury which is current/recurring or requires surgery)

Past History

Have you had . . .

Epilepsy	Yes ☐	No ☐
Diabetes	Yes ☐	No ☐
Heart Problems	Yes ☐	No ☐
Heart Murmur	Yes ☐	No ☐
Asthma/Bronchitis	Yes ☐	No ☐
Hernia	Yes ☐	No ☐
Concussion	Yes ☐	No ☐

Do you wear . . .

Glasses	Yes ☐	No ☐
Contact Lenses		
Soft	Yes ☐	No ☐
Hard	Yes ☐	No ☐
Protective Equipment	Yes ☐	No ☐
Mouth Guard		
at training	Yes ☐	No ☐
at competition	Yes ☐	No ☐
Other	Yes ☐	No ☐

If yes, please specify

Have you sustained . . .

A fracture in last 3 years Yes ☐ No ☐

If yes, where?

A dislocation   Yes ☐ No ☐

If yes, where?

Do you suffer from . . .

Recurring pain in any joint or muscle with play/practice?   Yes ☐ No ☐

If yes, where?

Back / Neck pain   Yes ☐ No ☐

Have you ever been treated for a head, neck or spinal injury?   Yes ☐   No ☐

Details

Does this condition affect your performance?

To the best of my knowledge, all information contained on this sheet is correct
(if under 18 please have parent or legal guardian sign)

Signature   Date

APPENDIX E

Useful sports medicine information resources for sports trainers

Organisation	Brief description	Web link
Australian Drug Foundation	Alcohol and drug information	www.adf.org.au
Australian Health Practitioner Regulation Agency	Information about registered health professionals and regulated medical practices	www.ahpra.gova.au
Australian Resuscitation Council	Peak body for first aid and CPR in Australia	www.resus.org.au
Australian Sport and Anti-Doping Agency	Information and rules about drugs in sport	www.asada.gov.au
CleanEdge	Sports Medicine Australia's CleanEdge is a website containing anti-doping, body image and overtraining information for participants, parents, teachers and coaches involved in sport, physical activity, recreation and fitness in the community	www.cleanedge.com.au
Food for Health	Dietary and healthy eating information	www.nhmrc.gov.au
Medical emergency planning: a practical guide for clubs	A planning guide and checklist that can be used to develop a medical emergency plan	www.smartplay.com.au
Play by the Rules	Information and online learning on discrimination, harassment and child abuse for the sport and recreation industry	www.playbytherules.com.au
Privacy Australia	Information about the National Privacy Principles, which includes rules on the collection and storage of medical records	www.privacy.gov.au
SmartPlay	Sports Medicine Australia's SmartPlay program promotes sports safety and injury prevention. The program aims to reduce the incidence and severity of sport and recreation injuries through the provision of evidence-based information and resources, guidelines and checklists	www.smartplay.com.au
Sports Dietitians Australia	Information including sports nutrition fact sheets	www.sportsdietitians.com.au
Sports Injury Tracker	SMA's online sports injury surveillance system developed for community sport, which enables data collection and analysis by club trainers and medical personnel	www.sportsinjurytracker.com.au
Sports Medicine Australia (SMA)	Information and resources about safe sport and physical activity	www.sma.org.au
World Anti Doping Agency	World governing body	www.wada-ama.org

GLOSSARY

abduction	Movement away from the midline of the body.
adduction	Movement towards the midline of the body.
AIDS	Acquired immunodeficiency syndrome.
anatomical position	The reference point for standard body position. The position resembles 'standing at attention', except the palms face forward and the thumbs point away from the body.
anterior	Nearer to the front of the body (e.g. the sternum is on the anterior side of the body).
AQF	Australian Qualifications Framework.
ASADA	Australian Sports Anti-Doping Authority.
avulsion (tooth)	Occurs when a permanent tooth is knocked out of the socket completely.
ballistic stretching	Stretching technique that uses repetitive bouncing motions.
bursa	A small sac of fibrous tissue lined with synovial fluid.
carbohydrate	Any one of a large group of compounds, including sugar and starch, which contain carbon, hydrogen and oxygen. Carbohydrates are important as a source of human energy.
cardiac muscle	Muscle found only in the heart and under automatic body control.
circumduction	The distal end of the bone follows a circular path and the proximal end stays stable. Circumduction is a combination of flexion, abduction, extension and adduction.
Concentric contraction	Shortening of a muscle.
contralateral	On the opposite side of the body (e.g. the spleen is contralateral to the liver).
contusion	A soft tissue injury affecting muscle tissue and blood vessels, which bleed into the muscle.
CPR	Cardiopulmonary resuscitation.
cyanosis	Bluish discolouration of the skin resulting from an inadequate amount of oxygen in the blood.
deep	Farther from the surface (e.g. the tendons are deep to the skin).
defibrillation	Administration of a controlled electric shock to restore normal heart rhythm.
depressants	Drugs that have the ability to slow down activity in the central nervous system. They have a calming and relaxing effect on the body in low doses and adversely affect coordination and concentration.
dietary fibre	A plant-based substance that is undigested by the body. Dietary fibre aids in the removal of unwanted chemicals from the intestine, prevents constipation, aids in weight control and helps to prevent intestinal cancers and control blood sugar and cholesterol levels.
dislocation	Displacement from the normal position of bones meeting at a joint.
distal	Farther from the body (e.g. the foot is distal to the hip).
dorsiflexion	Lifting the foot towards the shin.
DRSABCD	**D**anger, **R**esponsive?, **S**end for help, open **A**irway, normal **B**reathing?, commence **CPR**, attach **D**efibrillator.
EBV	Epstein-Barr virus.
eccentric contraction	Lengthening of a muscle while contracting.
EIA	Exercise-induced asthma.
eversion	Movement of the sole of the foot outwards.

Glossary

extension	Movement at a joint resulting in an increase in the angle between the two bones.
fats (lipids)	Substance containing one or more fatty acids and is one form in which energy is stored in the body.
flexion	Movement at a joint resulting in a decrease in the angle between the two bones.
fracture	Breakage of a bone, either complete or incomplete.
hallucinogenic (or psychedelic) drugs	Drugs that alter a person's perception of reality. They affect all the senses and can also markedly alter mood and thought.
HIV	Human immunodeficiency virus.
hypoglycaemia	Low blood sugar.
inadvertent doping	When an athlete uses a medication to treat an illness without realising that it contains a banned substance, and consequently returns a positive drug-test result.
inferior	Nearer to the soles of the feet (e.g. the liver is inferior to the heart).
insoluble fibre	Does not dissolve in water (e.g. whole grains, bran, corn).
inversion	Movement of the sole of the foot inwards.
ipsilateral	On the same side of the body (e.g. the gallbladder is ipsilateral to the liver).
isometric contraction	A contraction where there is no change in the length of the muscle or in the angle of the joint at which the contraction takes place.
lateral	Away from the midline (e.g. the ears are on the lateral side of the head).
ligament	A tough band of connective tissue that links two bones together at a joint.
luxation	Occurs when a tooth is loosened or pushed out of position.
medial	Nearer to the midline of the body (e.g. the heart is medial to the lungs).
metacarpophalangeal joint	Joint where the bones in the hand meet the bones in the fingers.
minerals	The basic chemical elements used in the body to help form body structures and regulate body processes.
mitochondria	A structure occurring in varying numbers inside the fluid of every cell. It is the site of the cell's energy production.
NO HARM principle	**H**eat, **A**lcohol, **R**unning, **M**assage.
NSAIDS	Non-steroidal anti-inflammatory drugs.
nutrition	The study of food in relation to the processes of the human body. The science of nutrition includes the study of diets and of the conditions resulting from a dietary deficiency.
plantar flexion	Pointing the foot.
PNF stretching	See proprioceptive neuromuscular facilitation stretching.
posterior	Nearer to the back of the body (e.g. the scapula is on the posterior side of the body).
pronation	Inward rotation of the forearm (palm faces posterior).
proprioceptive neuromuscular facilitation (PNF) stretching	Involves a combination of static and isometric muscle stretches in order to increase flexibility and prevent injury.
protein	Complex molecule made up of one or more amino acids and linked by peptide bonds. They form structural material of the human body including muscles, tissues, organs etc.
proximal	Nearer to the body (e.g. the shoulder is proximal to the hand).
RICER principle	**R**est, **I**ce, **C**ompression, **E**levation, **R**eferral.
rotation	Movement of a bone around its own axis. During rotation there should not be any other movement.
RPL	Recognition of prior learning.
SAMPLE principle	**S**igns and symptoms, **A**llergies, **M**edication, **P**ast history, **L**ast meal, **E**vent.

skeletal muscle	Tissue comprising the bulk of the body's muscle tissue. It is attached to the skeleton and is responsible for the movement of bones and voluntary muscles.
smooth muscle	Muscle found in the intestine and under automatic body control.
soluble fibre	Dissolves or swells in water (e.g., fruit and vegetables, oats, barley, legumes, psyllium husks).
SPF	Sun protection factor.
SPIED factors	**S**pecificity of the exercise, **P**articipants' energy levels, **I**ntensity of the exercise, **E**nvironmental conditions, **D**uration of the exercise.
static stretching	Passively stretching a muscle by placing it in a maximal stretch and holding it there.
stimulants	Drugs that have the ability to increase activity in the central nervous system. They often make a person feel more alert and confident but may also cause overstimulation.
STOP principle	**S**top, **T**alk, **O**bserve, **P**revent.
subluxation	Incomplete or partial dislocation.
superficial	Near to the surface or on the surface (e.g. the skin is superficial to muscle).
superior	Nearer to the top of the head (e.g. the eyes are superior to the mouth).
supination	Outward rotation of the forearm (palm faces anterior).
tendon	Tough whitish cord that serves to attach a muscle to a bone.
TOTAPS approach	**T**alk to the injured athlete, **O**bserve the injured area, **T**ouch the injured area, **A**ctive movement assessment, **P**assive movement assessment, **S**kills test.
ventilation	The passage of air into and out of the respiratory tract.
vitamins	Any of a group of substances that are required for healthy growth and development. They are divided into water soluble or fat soluble vitamins.
WADA	World Anti-Doping Agency.
WBGT	Wet Bulb Globe Temperature.

INDEX

Page numbers followed by 'f' indicate figures and 't' indicate tables.

Index

Index

Index